LIVE F
(OR AT LEAST TO 100)

LIVE FOREVER (OR AT LEAST TO 100)

MORE LIFE-SAVING STRATEGIES FROM TOM TASSEFF

THOMAS TASSEFF

*With Best Wishes to my
Long-time friend Tom
Considine for a longer,
healthier and happier life—*
Tom Tasseff
Dec. 27, 2017
Phone 716-646-3059

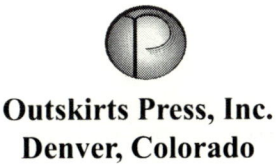

Outskirts Press, Inc.
Denver, Colorado

Live Forever (Or At Least to 100)
More Life-Saving Strategies From Tom Tasseff
All Rights Reserved.
Copyright © 2010 Thomas Tasseff
v2.0

The Author of:
Win the Ultimate Battle for your Health: The Lifesaving Legacy of Tom Tasseff

Cover Photo © 2010 JupiterImages Corporation. All rights reserved - used with permission.

Outskirts Press, Inc.
http://www.outskirtspress.com

PB ISBN: 978-1-4327-6240-7

Library of Congress Control Number: 2010931064

Outskirts Press and the "OP" logo are trademarks belonging to Outskirts Press, Inc.

PRINTED IN THE UNITED STATES OF AMERICA

I wish to express my sincere gratitude
and dedicate this book to my dear wife, Nada,
to my three children, Clint, Maria, and Alexandra,
and to my seven grandchildren,
Athan, Athena, Paul, Holly, Andrew, Nicholas, and Alexis.
I further dedicate this book to the 175 million Americans
who will so needlessly die of cancer and other horrible
but entirely preventable diseases in the near future
Finally, I dedicate this book to the 300 million living Americans
who will sadly lose so many loved ones in the next few years,
but who can do something to prevent these horrible deaths
by living longer, healthier, and happier lives...
Beginning right now!
It is You to whom I dedicate this book...
My Legacy to You!

Other Books by Tom Tasseff:
Win the Ultimate Battle for Your Health:
The Lifesaving Legacy of Tom Tasseff.
Outskirts Press: Denver, Colorado. 2008. 236 Pages.

Contents

Preface

This book was written in my eightieth year of life to share with you new information that has come to light since the publication of my first book, *Win the Ultimate Battle for Your Health: The Lifesaving Legacy of Tom Tasseff* (Outskirts Press 2008; Amazon.com; Barnes & Noble). Although each book stands alone perfectly well in its respective lifesaving strategies, I strongly recommend that you obtain a copy of my earlier work at once and keep both of these books in your arsenal of lifesaving literature. Together they provide you the means to a longer, happier, and healthier life… my continuing legacy to you!

My intention in writing this book is to share with you what I have learned and employed in winning the ultimate battle for my own health as based upon a lifetime of good living, from conducting my own in-depth research, and from the experience of overcoming my own health obstacles. My legacy to you is to provide you with the ammunition that I have found available and have used to improve my own general health and happiness.

It is my hope that as you read this book, you will do so with an open mind and find both the information and the inspiration to continue to do your own research, to seek appropriate and cooperative professional medical health care consultation as necessary, and to make informed decisions that will lead you to a healthier and happier life.

None of the information provided nor any of the opinions expressed in this publication should be construed as personal medical advice or instruction. No action should be taken based solely upon on the contents of this book. Readers are advised to consult their own appropriate health care professionals on any matters relating to their personal medical health, health concerns, symptoms, illness, disease, or treatment strategies. This means… "See Your Doctor."

No information contained herein, as expressed, or as implied, or as might be interpreted by the reader, is intended to diagnose, treat, cure, or prevent any disease. That is why the reader is advised again to seek his or her own personal professional medical consultation.

I have done my very best to ensure that the contents of this book are accurate. The information contained herein is based upon my own personal research and personal experience and while I believe it to be correct and accurate as based entirely upon my own research and experience, it cannot be guaranteed in any way to be correct and accurate. No warrantee or guarantee of any kind is stated, intended, expressed, or implied.

While the information provided and the opinions expressed in this book are believed to be accurate and are based on the best judgment of the author, readers who fail to consult with appropriate health care authorities assume ALL risk for ANY injury and for consequences of any kind.

Neither the author, nor the publisher, nor any person or persons associated with the writing, editing, publication, printing, or distribution of this book is liable for any errors, inaccuracies, or omissions. The reader assumes ALL responsibility for ANY actions taken and is repeatedly advised to seek appropriate professional medical consultation.

Neither the U.S. Food and Drug Administration (USFDA) nor the American Medical Association (AMA) have approved any of the materials contained, practices described, or information presented in this book. The author does however recommend that the USFDA, the AMA, medicine, big medicine, big drug and pharmaceutical companies, and big money finally admit to us the benefits of natural and herbal remedies, which can quickly and cost effectively save millions of our dollars and both prolong and save millions of our lives each year.

Acknowledgements

I do not believe that it would have been possible to write this book without the thoughtful and persistent encouragement of my granddaughter, Holly Kubicki who graduated from The State University of New York College at Buffalo in 2007 with honors and is now a certified secondary school Mathematics teacher in New York. She has recently received her Masters Degree and has, along with all of my children and grandchildren made us very proud.

Holly helped me to realize that my lifetime accumulation of health and fitness knowledge should be shared with others so that they too might benefit from all of the things that have contributed to my longevity, good health, and happiness. She was instrumental in the preparation of the early drafts of the manuscript, which has now become this book.

I have been very fortunate while writing this book to have such a friend as Steven J. Wamback who did the technical and manual editing of several versions of the manuscript and skillfully guided its progress toward publication and greater public appeal. Having graduated from The State University of New York College at Fredonia, New York with degrees in both the Geological and Biological Sciences, Steve has worked as a biologist, geologist, and environmental scientist on various projects within the realms of natural resource conservation; biomedical research and science publication; technical project writing and editing; and public education. Steve finds himself at home with his family in Angola, New York on the beautiful shores of Lake Erie where he enjoys fossil hunting, sausage making, astronomy, and amateur radio when time permits.

Chapter 1
Chronic Inflammation and Relief from Muscular and Joint Pain

The Human body was designed by God through billions of years of evolution and under the pressure of Natural Selection to last indefinitely in a state of strength, health, and unlimited productivity... assuming, of course, that we take good care of it. The longer and the better we take good care of our bodies, the longer we will live. Old age is merely the cumulative result of illness and disease.

Practically everything that conventional doctors have been taught about disease, illness, health, and nutrition is largely incorrect. Doctors have never cured anyone's disease or illness and neither have their medicines. Our immune system is the only thing that we have that keeps us in good health and free of illness and disease.

All diseases and illnesses are caused by toxins, parasites, yeasts, viruses, fungi, and bacteria... all of, which we have been carrying with us since the day we were born. Throughout our childhood, these invasive organisms, parasites, and their toxins have been responsible for any and all of our various diseases and illnesses. As we became adults, invasive organisms continued to multiply, which lead to more adult-onset illnesses and diseases. Ultimately, they will be the cause of our death, unless we take immediate measures to eliminate them.

The only way we can achieve this potential is to eliminate the invaders and their by-products through a healthy and well-maintained immune system... an immune system that actively has been kept fully charged, strong, and efficient.

A review of recent articles published between 2002 and the present in both popular and scientific literature indicates that various forms of chronic inflammation attract major attention in the medical world. Nature's way of telling us that something is going wrong in our body is most often revealed to us via some form of chronic inflammation.

One of the first things that medical students are taught is to be ever mindful of the four cardinal signs of inflammation... *rubor, calor, tumor,* and *dolar*... Latin words for redness, heat, swelling, and pain.

It is important for us to know and understand that inflammation is our body's basic defense against invasive organisms, toxins, and disease. The process of inflammation begins with some triggering event such as a virus, bacteria, parasite, or any number of toxins invading the body; or merely by eating harmful junk food; or from physical injuries such as cuts, falls, and surgeries.

In order to get to the root of any pain, it is necessary to find out what is triggering the inflammation in our body and then to take the proper action to stop it. Inflammation is the body's natural response to something that is wrong such as infection, open cut injuries, or tissue destruction anywhere (or somewhere) in the body.

It is also the inflammatory response that triggers the remainder of our self-defensive immune system to begin to solve the problem by sending white cells (macrophages) to attack various offenders such as bacteria, viruses, pollutants, toxins, chemicals, trans-fatty acids, physical irritants, injuries, hormonal imbalances, and many others. Macrophages surround foreign bodies (antigens) with their foot like-pseudopodia just like the amoebas you saw engulfing food under the microscope in your high school biology class. If you recall, the name of this particle engulfing process was phagocytosis.

Once the inflammation process is triggered, white cells (macrophages) rush to the affected area and produce pro-inflammatory chemical messengers (cytokines) to attack and clean up (consume and digest) the cells in the affected area. If the inflammatory trigger is not stopped, the pro-inflammatory chemical messengers (cytokines) continue to rise and possibly destroy more cells, which will eventually lead to organ damage. When the injury or offending problem is eliminated, the body's normal response is to stop or slow down the inflammation process as the infected area is cleaned up.

Older people do not eliminate or reduce the inflammation process as efficiently as younger people do. In some cases of the elderly, their bodies lose their ability to stop the pro-inflammatory response until excess tissue destruction becomes a serious disease. If the inflammation continues, we experience more destruction and chronic inflammation. This ultimately causes our immune system to become over-stimulated and unregulated. This leads to increasing degrees of redness, heat, swelling, and pain and further inflammatory autoimmune problems such as arthritis and fibromyalgia.

As far back as the early 1990's Dr. Paul Ridker, a cardiologist at Brigham and Women's Hospital, and the father of modern inflammation research, was convinced that cholesterol was not causing plaque in the arteries to burst and cause heart attacks, but that some sort of inflammatory reaction was responsible. In a cover article in *Time* magazine (February 2004), Dr. Ridker said, "Just a few short years ago, nobody was interested in this stuff. Now, the whole field of inflammation research is about to explode. Inflammation is the body's first defense against infection, but when it goes wrong, it can lead to heart attacks, colon cancer, Alzheimer's and a host of other diseases."

Dr. Andrew Weil is a leading integrative medicine specialist and respected health and wellness advocate who says, "Chronic Inflammation just may be the root of ALL degenerative disease."

In the year 2000, the prestigious *New England Journal of Medicine* published several studies that showed high levels of chronic inflammation signal significantly greater risk for heart attack, stroke, and Alzheimer's disease.

In February 2002, the leading medical journal on cancer, *Oncology,* published a landmark study, "Chronic Inflammation and Cancer" in which it reported, "A substantial body of evidence supports the conclusion that chronic inflammation can predispose individuals to cancer. The longer the inflammation persists, the higher the risk."

Our immune system, eighty percent of which lies within our intestinal tract, relies heavily upon enzymes in order to perform its defensive function fighting off the agents that cause inflammation.

Enzymes are specialized protein molecules manufactured by living organisms and which function as biological catalysts. Catalysts are molecules, elements, and compounds that speed up chemical reactions to rates greater than merely due to chance. Although these reactions would eventually occur anyway, enzymatic catalysis directs biological processes and causes these reactions to occur fast enough to allow life to exist. We might accurately think of catalysts and enzymes as "chemical matchmakers."

There are three classes of enzymes in our bodies: metabolic enzymes, which run our bodies; digestive enzymes, which digest our food; and food enzymes, which are taken in from raw food (other organisms that we consume) and which help start food digestion. There are more than 3,000 active enzymes at work in our body combining with co-enzymes, directing, coordinating, and speeding up 100,000 chemical reactions… ensuring proper functioning of our bodies, maintaining our good health, and keeping us alive.

Enzymes are fascinating. Enzymatic systems make up essential components of the normal functioning of ALL living things. They, like all proteins, consist of chains of amino acids formed under the direct supervision of RNA (ribonucleic acid) according to the template laid out by DNA (deoxyribonucleic acid), the blueprint for life which occurs in the form of chromosomes in nucleus of each of our cells.

These specialized protein molecules are responsible for directing, modifying, accelerating, or retarding all body functions. Enzymes are the body's labor force used to perform every function needed for our daily activities and are required in keeping us alive. They are responsible for every function of every organ system in the human body... including our body's inflammatory response to injury or invasion as well as our sustained immune response to effectively rid our bodies of the causal pathogens or toxic agents.

In addition to this important function supporting our immune system, enzymes are also required in the digestion, absorption, and metabolism of food and nutrients. Enzymes also enable us to see, smell, taste, hear, breathe, and move. They are also required for cardiovascular functions, blood coagulation system, liver, kidneys, elimination of toxins, excretion, reproduction and more. If enzyme activity stops, life stops and the person (or any living organism) eventually dies.

Therefore, it is important for us to eat natural whole foods that contain live enzymes, co-enzymes, vitamins, minerals and amino acid constituents to help maintain a healthy supply of all of our essential enzymes. Whenever our bodies are injured or when we sustain any type of injury due to a cut or bruise, under enzymatic control, the protein fibrin forms a thin very hard protective mesh coating around the affected area. As our wounds heal, the fibrin net dissipates by reabsorption to bring the affected area back to normal.

When we have chronic aches or pains anywhere throughout our body's muscles or bone joints, many of the most popular pain medications only give temporary relief by treating the inflammation, which is only a symptom of the problem. They do no target the actual cause of the problem.

As soon as our body senses an injury or any sudden change of temperature, it reacts by sending white cells to the injury site to fight the infection, thereby causing inflammation and swelling. At this time, fibrin is also released as a protective mesh around the injury site, which also stops the bleeding in cuts and bruises.

Ordinarily, when healing takes place and things return to normal, the fibrin breaks down and the inflammation disappears. Frequently, however, the inflammation remains and the fibrin never breaks down and continues around the site. It also continues to harden and cause more inflammation and excruciating pain remains, as we approach middle age.

Research indicates inflammation is less likely to dissipate if we are over 50 years of age because your bodies lack the necessary enzymes, which normally dissolve the fibrin. Since many of us are deficient in these enzymes, we remain suffering with unrelenting and unbearable pain in various parts of our bodies. Arthritis and fibromyalgia are two prime examples of this chronic source of pain.

Researchers have discovered a naturally occurring compound, which many consider a "Miracle Enzyme". Taken in pill form, this enzyme helps to get rid of the old fibrin molecular net responsible for inflammation and pain. It is called serrapeptase (AKA serratiopeptase / serratiopepti-dase). It dissolves clots and fibrin nets allowing blood to flow freely again. The redness, heat, swelling, and pain of inflammation are thereby relieved.

Most enzymes eventually lose their potency and they ultimately become depleted. This decrease occurs over time and is due to combinations of advancing age, poor nutrition, and failing health. This process of decreasing enzyme activity begins as early as the age of 27 but it generally begins at about 40 years of age or so.

Serrapeptase cuts through any fibrin mesh and allows our joints and muscles to move without stress or pain. It is very effective in relieving pain due to: Arthritis, Aching Knees, Joint Pain, Lower Back and General Back Pains, Muscular Aches, Discomfort of Hips, Fibromyalgia, Swollen Joints and Aching Bones, Swollen Ankles, Swollen Feet, Swollen Fingers, Swollen Legs and Knees, Pinched Nerves, Sprains, Carpel Tunnel Syndrome, Tendonitis, Rheumatism, Bursitis, Sciatica, Shingles, Whiplash, Sports Injuries, Inflammation of the veins and many others.

Since our chronic pain problems accumulated over time, we should also allow the serrapeptase some time to do its job properly. One might begin to notice results in 2 to 3 weeks. Some people notice results in as little as a few days.

About 3.7 million Americans suffer from the

unrelenting pain of fibromyalgia. Some days they wake up with aches all over their body, which never go away leaving them exhausted and stressed. Even the strongest pain medications do not seem to help.

According to the Life Extension Foundation, over 140 studies have established that high levels of fibrin and chronic inflammation predict significantly greater risk for serious disease and death. Serrapeptase has been shown to significantly reduce both fibrin and inflammation.

Dr. William Wong became a fibromyalgia [FMS] patient in 1990 and then began his search to make his workday easier. He soon realized that fibromyalgia was due to over-deposition of fibrin.

Dr. Wong worked many months to find an effective treatment for fibrin overload related to fibromyalgia, during that time this painful condition was wracking his body. He eventually found the solution and wanted to share it with the rest of the world. He stated in his own words, "I believe it is a moral imperative that this multi-dimensional approach and its rationale be shared with the rest of the health care community."

Dr. Wong's solution included the proteolytic enzyme serrapeptase. It cracks away the hard fibrin meshes and frees our bodies from excruciating pain thereby allowing us to move about more freely and to live completely without pain.

In order to fight inflammation and to remove the unhealthy levels of fibrin, protein-eating enzymes or prote-olytic enzymes (proteases) in serrapepdase are necessary to devour the excess fibrin. Proteases are the enzymes responsible for increasing breakdown of the fibrin build-up, which is in turn composed of structural proteins (Re-member the enzyme-containing detergent commercials on television which for years informed us that, "Protein gets out protein.") Serrapepdase also helps create Plasmins, the fibrin-eating enzymes in our blood plasma, which dis-solve clotting factors especially in the bloodstream itself or upon the healing of injuries when the blood clot is no longer needed.

We each have our very own fountain of youth within each of our bodies; and we can maintain its maximum per-formance by increasing our intake of enzymes that keep it functioning. Excessive amounts of fibrin can cause blood clot formation that may block a coronary artery and can cause a heart attack or block a cerebral artery leading to a stroke. *Life Extension Magazine* reports that the use of most drugs dealing with cholesterol does nothing to break down fibrin that actually may be closing our arteries. By taking aggressive preventative actions, we can dramati-cally reduce our chances of dying from cardiovascular disease.

According to many studies, serrapeptase can reduce in-flammation, lower cholesterol, and break up blood clots to prevent disasters of the heart and brain such as heart attacks or strokes. *The Journal of International Medicine* reported that serrapeptase prevents fluid retention and swelling in our tissues by conferring anti-inflammatory properties. It is superior to other related anti-inflammatory enzymes.

Some researchers believe that hidden inflammation could be responsible for causing Heart Attack, Stroke, Colon Disease, Alzheimer's, and many others. Even when inflammation occurs after stubbing a toe or getting a splinter in a finger our risk for other immune response related diseases increases. Evidence is mounting which is changing physician's ideas of what actually makes us sick.

Serrapeptase is a completely all-natural product that has anti-fibrin properties, anti-pain and anti-swelling features with no side effects. Serrapeptase helps with all sorts of pain and has a 40-year history of helping with all sorts of pain. It can immediately end our pain regardless of where the pain is or how long we have suffered with it.

Inflammation and the rest of our immune system's response to it has become one of the most important areas of current medical research. Medical publications are reporting new ways each month that chronic inflammation harms the body by destabilizing cholesterol deposits in the coronary arteries and leading to heart attacks and strokes. It also harms the nerve cells in the brains of Alzheimer's disease victims.

Instead of using complex alternate unnatural treatment options, this very intriguing concept employing a more natural option brings to the forefront a new and possibly simpler way of preventing and mitigating disease. A single inflammation-reducing remedy could possibly prevent heart disease, strokes, colon disease, and Alzheimer's disease. By reducing inflammation, Serrapeptase reduces the pain and the inflammation by blocking the release of pain inducing amines from inflamed tissues. Thus, the cycle of pain and inflammation is broken.

Unless we first get rid of excess and unnecessary fibrin deposits, whether it is in our muscles, bones, veins, or arteries, healing and return to normal health cannot begin. Excessive amounts of fibrin build up in our tissues and can cause all types of pain, or even the onset of certain painless diseases such as cholesterol-related plaque deposits, hardening of the arteries (atherosclerosis), a host of cancers, and many other diseases.

Chapter 2
Human Growth Hormone
(The Fountain of Youth)

During the late fifties, the Russian physician Dr. Vladimir Dillman proposed that our bodies have an internal hormonal clock in the pituitary gland, which is the "Master Gland" of our endocrine system and is located in the hypothalamus area of the brainstem. He also believed that a change in hormone balance resulted in the aging of the body and if this balance could be improved, it could slow down the aging process, and may even reverse it. Human Growth Hormone (HGH) is considered the most important of these hormones.

The depletion of Human Growth Hormone (HGH) affects every cell in our body and thereby is responsible for degeneration and aging. The pituitary gland produces Human Growth Hormone (HGH), which we normally have in abundance. We released it easily during our youth but as we age, the pituitary gland does not release it so easily any longer.

Medical Science once believed that Human Growth Hormone (HGH) was needed only while the body grew into maturity, then the hormone was not necessary any longer. However, research and further studies have revealed that HGH is vital to all bodily functions throughout the life cycle and even into our old age. Research has also revealed that our body's release of HGH tends to diminish as maturity is reached. It has been suggested that HGH levels could be reduced by up to 80 percent between ages 20 and 60. Since HGH levels diminish as we age, the proper functioning of many of our organs is compromised and this contributes further to the aging process.

Regardless of our current age, we can achieve new vigor and vitality and maintain it well into the future. We can melt off fat, increase muscle mass, increase endurance, restore hair growth, improve skin tone, boost sexual response, and boost our immune systems. We can also take 20 years off our age without injections, drugs, synthetic hormones, side effect, stressful exercise, or diets.

According to Dr. Daniel Rudman (1990), "Studies indicate HGH deficiency is relevant to health and responsible for early onset of degenerative disease, or even premature death."

Somatotropin is another name for the Human Growth Hormone (HGH) produced in the pituitary on command by the hypothalamus gland. The anti aging magic of HGH occurs mostly at night during our sleep.

HGH could be the most important discovery in recent years, which affects our body's aging process. Results of experiments with HGH by Dr. Daniel Rudman were reported in the *New England Journal of Medicine* in 1990. The reported results were over a six-month period among a group of men between the ages of 61 to 81 and reported to have reversed their biological age by 10 to 20 years. Thousands of additional studies have been performed throughout the world documenting that HGH retards aging and actually reverses the aging process throughout the whole body.

Dr. Edmund Chein, MD, directed a study at Palm Springs Life Extension by increasing HGH levels with low doses of frequent HGH injections, which proved to be 100 percent effective on all of his patients. Some of Dr. Chein's assessed effects upon sizable percentages of his patients include:

Decreased Body Fat	72%
Increased Muscle Size	81%
Increased Muscle Strength	88%
Increased Exercise Tolerance	81%
Increased Exercise Endurance	83%,

Improved Skin Thickness	68%
Improved Skin Texture and Elasticity	69%
Increased Wrinkle Disappearance	51%
Increased New Hair Growth	38%
Increased Healing Capacity	71%
Increased Resistance to Common Illness	73%
Increased Energy Level	84%
Improved Emotional Stability	67%
Improved Attitude toward Life	78%
Improved Memory	62%
Improved Sexual Potency and Frequency	75%
Improved Duration of Penile Erection	62%
Decreased Frequency of Night Time Urination	52%
Decreased Hot Flashes in Menopause	58%
Improved Menstrual Cycle Regulation	38%

Increased Bone Density and many other improvements.

These fantastic results were achieved with HGH injections at a cost of about $1,000 per month, which would be well out of reach for the average person.

A better, cheaper, faster, and easier way to gain benefits of HGH therapy came about in 1997 when Dr. L. E. Dorman made a remarkable presentation before the American College for the Advancement of Medicine. He revealed that HGH production declines after age 30 and rapidly declines to speed up aging and that the body's ability to release the HGH is compromised. His research concluded that it was not necessary to give painful injections into the body with all of its side effects or the price tag of $1,000 a month. Instead of this method, a natural method was needed to release the body's own natural HGH.

Doctors Dorman and Marsh have identified Growth Hormone Releasers, called secretagogue compounds. These natural compounds consisting of amino acids, proteins and botanical extracts enhance the body's production of HGH and help to release and utilize it. No matter how old we are, secretagogues do this with their amazing super nutrients in a stacked amino acid complex of protein fragments, peptides, and complex polysaccharides that stimulate receptors in the pituitary and hypothalamus glands to help release the body's stores of growth hormone.

Medical research indicates that this induced release mechanism for natural HGH could mimic the body's youthful secretory mechanism of HGH release better than administration of some other available sources of HGH.

The natural growth hormone is not contained in the growth hormone releaser secretagogue because it functions by stimulating the body to secrete its own stores of natural HGH. This new miracle of HGH release (secretagogues) can help us to live longer, healthier and happier lives. Secretagogues are safe, powerful, and much less expensive than the possible $1,000 per month cost of painful injections and associated side effects.

Dr. Marsh believes, "In many situations, secretagogues

are not only as effective as an HGH injection, but they also have other distinct advantages."

If after the age of 35, we have a desire to maintain our appearance and biological age as long as possible, we can start taking HGH. During our early hours of sleep, small pulses of HGH are secreted and stay in circulation for only a few short minutes until the liver quickly absorbs the HGH and begins to metabolize it. Human Growth Hormone truly is a fountain of youth.

Chapter 3
The Immune System

Science reveals that 70 to 85 percent of our immune cells occur within our gut (gastrointestinal tract) where 80 trillion bacteria also reside in cozy comfort. One might wonder about the 80 trillion bacteria in our gut versus the 70 to 100 trillion cells in our body. The reason is that the bacteria are hundreds of times smaller than our body cells.

Our digestive systems serve as homes to as many as 500 different types of bacteria, 85% friendly (probiotic) and 15% unfriendly (antibiotic). Friendly bacteria in our gut stimulate our body's vital immune system by increasing the production of immune enhancing substances like IgA, one of our immune system's Immunoglobulin Antibodies, but this ratio can reverse itself with time.

Our resident intestinal bacteria are composed of 100 to 400 different species, which establish themselves and make themselves at home in our intestines. They have essentially become part of us, through co-evolution and symbiosis in which both they and we receive advantages from their presence.

These friendly bacteria are the so-called probiotics we hear so much about these days and are our first line of immune system defense. They support our immune systems by neutralizing carcinogenic substances and help to suppress tumors that might happen to occur in our intestines. Certain harmful species of bacteria that can also occur within us cause constipation, diarrhea, injury to our intestines, and can lead to intestinal tumors.

As we age, we harbor fewer of the good bacteria, because of our widespread use of antibiotics. Even if we are not personally aware of taking antibiotics, we actually are! It has been reported that over 35 million pounds of antibiotics are produced each year in the United States. Most of these are given to poultry, pigs, and cattle routinely to prevent infections and diseases in their stressful environments.

Because of this preponderance of antibiotics in use and in addition to their occurring in our food, they are beginning to show up in our lakes, rivers, and drinking water supplies as well. Therefore, when we ingest food or water from any of these sources, we are also ingesting antibiotics.

Antibiotics are non-selectively detrimental to our good bacteria as well as to our bad bacteria. To add further insult to injury, all of this intentional and unintentional use of antibiotics is evolving increasingly antibiotic resistant strains of bacteria such that super-antibiotic-resistant bacteria have become problematic and are getting worse.

Stress, medications, and poor diet also reduce the healthy bacteria in our gastrointestinal tracts, which leaves us susceptible to infections and diseases that arise from overworked immune systems. Even though many types of prescription drugs can be responsible for this decrease, the most common cause of decreased healthy intestinal flora is the use of antibiotics.

About 85 percent of the bacteria in our gut are beneficial provided that we have healthy digestive systems. As recently as the past few years, scientists began finding out that our sick intestines are causing a national health disaster.

Science has recently revealed that healthy bacterial cells in our digestive system help us to digest our food, boost our immune systems, control yeasts, parasites, and harmful bacteria, all of which can cause excessive gas, ulcers, and even food poisoning along with many other diseases. It has been revealed that about 85% of Americans are currently affected by human parasites. We share our bodies with a large number and a great variety of these invasive creatures.

Only about 132 species of parasites have been positively identified among the thousands of parasites that can possibly infect us. For people between 45 and 65 years of age, digestive problems of one type or another have become the second most common reason for hospitalization. This can be attributed to parasitic bacterial toxification, which generally increases with advancing age.

If the intestinal lining is damaged, it becomes more permeable and proper nutrients are no longer absorbed. Under these circumstances, our immune system can no longer protect us from bad bacteria, viruses, parasites, toxins, yeasts and certain large protein molecules that enter the bloodstream causing the body to treat them as foreign invaders, thereby triggering both inflammatory and auto-immune responses.

This increased intestinal permeability is referred to as the "Leaky Gut Syndrome". There are junctions or small spaces in the small intestinal lining between the cells that can open and close to appropriately allow larger or smaller molecules to pass. At times, these spaces become excessively large and allow toxins and large protein molecules to leak from the intestines into the bloodstream, where they are not desired.

If the immune system cells in our digestive tract do not

detoxify the toxins to which we are exposed on a daily basis and allow them to pass into our bloodstreams, then our livers cannot eliminate them safely from our bodies either; and the liver soon becomes overburdened. Therefore, toxins will build up and continue to circulate leading to inflammation and damage throughout the body, which can eventually develop into food allergies, sensitivities, and possible inflammatory damage throughout the entire body.

Since antibodies are produced in order to fight off any foreign invading particles that get into various body tissues, an inflammatory reaction can be triggered. Eventually, even more antibodies are produced, thereby causing chronic inflammation in that area.

A standard test for "Leaky Gut Syndrome" can be performed by your doctor using 'The Lactulose/Mannitol Test' to determine if you have a hyper-permeable intestine. The test consists of ingesting 5 grams of lactulose sugar and 5 grams of mannitol sugar. Leaky gut will be determined by the amount absorbed or excreted. This test is important for all Arthritic patients.

Daily or frequent use of foods rich in probiotic bacteria is the best way to protect our intestinal linings and to make sure that we maintain a strong and healthy colony of good bacteria. Pain medications, antibiotics, steroids and stress can destroy our natural good bacteria. Therefore, taking a powerful probiotic supplement of at least 15 billion cells with 12 to 16 multiple strains to support our intestinal integrity should also improve our health.

Probiotics can help prevent overgrowth of bad bacteria, yeasts, and parasites in the small and large intestines that lead to toxins in the body and which can eventually cause chronic inflammation.

If medications kill off the good bacteria, the bad yeasts (certain funguses such as Candida species) grow into fungal colonies, which can penetrate the intestinal lining and enter the bloodstream. In effect, this may cause serious infections and inflammation to joints and muscles. Even if prescription antifungal medications kill the fungus, the yeast overgrowth may reoccur if powerful supplementation is not followed up with regular use of probiotics.

Chapter 4
Epicor and the Immune System

I n 2005, it was discovered that a majority of the production floor workers in a small animal food factory
outside of Cedar Rapids, Iowa, were not using up any of
their available sick days. The insurance premiums at the
factory remained flat over several years, which in these
times of over inflated everything, is very unusual.

An investigation took place to help determine what
kept these workers exceptionally healthy. Blood samples
were taken from veteran production floor workers who
were producing a special animal feed additive derived
from yeast revealed that they had a much greater immune
response.

It was apparent that prolonged daily exposure to the

factory's yeast derivative products had turned the workers bodies into fortresses of immunity. The employees handling the yeast had caused their health insurance costs to decrease because they were taking fewer sick days.

This unexpected streak of good-health was attributed to the workers inadvertently inhaling small amounts of dust from the yeast, which was shown to enhance the employees' immune response and was thereby helping them to remain unusually healthy.

Researchers soon identified the immune boosting components from the yeast. Certain yeast derivatives were then sent to be specially processed, refined, and concentrated. Research efforts expanded quickly, which created the improved, concentrated form for Humans now known as "EpiCor".

Our white blood cells are especially active when foreign matter or bacterial cells invade our bodies. Two of our body's array of white blood cell types include T-Helper cells and T-Killer cells. When a disease-causing pathogen triggers an immune response, our body's T-Helper cells gather up and activate T-Killer cells. If the helper cells are properly nourished, they act quickly to deliver orders telling T-Killer cells where to attack the pathogen.

EpiCor effectively activates our entire immune response with the combination of 18 immune system supporting compounds, metabolites, and phytonutrients. This just might very well be the "Holy Grail" of immune system boosters.

Our immune system is much more complex than our white blood cells (macrophages) that attack invading germs. Immune-boosting metabolites and phytonutrients combine to activate our entire immune system.

B cells are stimulated to transport some of our white cells and increase the IgA cells in our intestinal tract area and help get rid of the undesired invaders. It also increases NK (Natural Killer) cell activity in order to help eliminate our body's own deformed and harmful cells.

EpiCor is such a powerful immune system enhancer that the number of white blood cells (macrophages), immune-boosting granulocytes, and NK cells reportedly increased dramatically in only two hours, during one study. EpiCor balances our immune system without over-stimulating our bodies and is safe to take it on a daily basis.

It would be very beneficial to also include a supplement of vitamin D, since our immune system's cells contain receptors for vitamin D to allow them to function properly. Studies have shown that vitamin D has a strong link to the immune system.

Our body manufactures vitamin D from sunlight. Therefore, most of us become deficient in appropriate concentrations of this vitamin during the winter months and vitamin D supplements should, in most cases, be taken.

Selenium in the form of selenomethionine should also be taken with EpiCor to enhance the immune system and to give our bodies the ultimate defense system. Selenomethionine can reach our muscle tissue, liver tissue and blood more efficiently than any other selenium product.

Selenium may help to maintain healthy DNA against aging and environmental factors. It favorably impacts genes that are linked to the progression of cancer. It also blasts oxidative stress by virtue of its antioxidant power.

Chapter 5
Lectinology and the Immune System

W e usually do not pay attention to our intestinal health until we develop an obvious gastrointestinal (GI) disease. Our bodies have 70 to 100 trillion cells working together in harmony to sustain our existence and our gastrointestinal tract is a critical component and it is one of the main barriers to the outside world of contaminates (pesticides, heavy metals, herbicides, lectins and more) that enter our bodies via the foods that we eat. Therefore, if we take probiotics, we are fortifying our GI tracts and enhancing the ability for nutrients from food and supplements to be more readily absorbed.

Celiac disease is an autoimmune disorder caused by the intolerance of wheat gluten. Recent research indicates that the lectin wheat germ agglutinin (WGA) causes allergic reactions in the gut, which release inflammatory cytokines and histamines linked to allergic reactions. Other studies show lectins increase gut permeability and obstruct digestion.

WGA has been identified as the major cause of rheumatoid arthritis. When this lectin leaves our intestine and enters our bloodstream, it eventually goes to the glycoconjugates in our connective tissue. When it arrives at this point, its bonds are strong and this directly contributes to the cause of arthritis-related joint stiffness.

WGA also helps to make us fat and helps to keep us fat. It mimics insulin by binding to our insulin receptors, which in turn stimulates indefinite production of fat in our cells. More recent research also shows frightening indications that these lectins are possibly linked in causing the worsening of autism. Even though wheat lectins are the largest problem, many different lectins cause their own types of health problems.

It can take thousands and even up to millions of cells to be sufficiently damaged in our body, before a problem is perceived. In order for the body to heal and to be healthy, toxic waste should be minimized. Annually, about 14 million people are hospitalized with GI problems including cancers and of which about 234,000 people die.

Our large intestine is approximately 5 feet in length with four segments, the 8 inches of ascending colon; 18

inches of transverse colon; about 12 inches of descending colon; and 18 inches of sigmoid colon.

When the large intestine receives water content from the small intestine, about 90 percent of it is absorbed. When food material and moisture are in the colon too long, the excess moisture is absorbed with toxins and waste being reabsorbed out of proportion and irritates the colon's lining.

This contributes to individuals failing to have 2 to 3 bowel movements per day, feeling ill and tired. This causes their stools to be harder and drier, because the body has re-absorbed the toxic wastewater. This process of absorption and reabsorption should encourage the daily nourishment of the GI tract, even when we are not experiencing any GI problems.

If we have a healthy intestinal lining, it is a selective barrier that only allows the properly digested proteins, starches and digested fats to cross over and enter the bloodstream. The mucosa is a single layer of epithelial cells lining the colon that regenerates every 3-8 days. This nutrient-dependent barrier must be properly maintained for sufficient healing, repair, and regeneration.

Diffusion is the process of nutrient absorption such as magnesium, potassium, sodium and free fatty acids through the intestinal cells. 'Active Transport' allows fatty acids, amino acids, glucose, vitamins and minerals to cross through cells.

The third way that substances can pass from the intestines into the circulatory system is through the tight junction spaces between cells lining the intestines that are normally sealed. If the intestinal lining becomes irritated from un-digestible herbicides, pesticides, heavy metals, antibiotics or other undesirables, the junctions become loose and begin to allow unwanted larger molecules in the intestines such as un-digestible vegetable lectins to pass through and into the blood.

This immediately triggers damage and immune system reactions because these larger molecules are recognized as foreign. Eventually, damage progresses to the intestinal lining and allows disease - causing bacteria, undigested food particles, and toxins to pass directly into the body. A series of events causes the immune system to become more involved in generating antibodies and cytokines that produce oxidative damage, localized irritation, and inflammation throughout the body.

Lectinology research is an extensive and emerging science that has far reaching implications and is still in its infancy. Scientific research reveals diseases appear to be brought on by an immune disorder caused by lectins. One example is the devastating autoimmune disorder referred to as Celiac Disease, affecting one out of every 133 people, which is brought on by our body's intolerance to the lectin called Wheat Germ Agglutin, presently existing in all wheat and grain products. I will try to explain lectins in the best way possible to break down complicated biological processes into easy-to-understand-English.

Lectins are a specialized class of proteins that are not degradable by the stomach or its enzymes. They are found in plants as part of their immune system and are commonly found in foods such as: grains, seeds, beans, nuts, some vegetables and fruits, and sea food. Many other foods contain lectins but the amounts of lectins present are not as high or potentially toxic. Virtually, all foods contain lectins. Some are our friends; others are neutral; others may be our enemies.

The effects of lectins are complex to understand due to our unique genetic make-up and state of health that also determines, which lectins that we are sensitive to and how we will react to them. Lectin damage can accumulate and not show up for years later in other parts of our bodies.

Every day, we consume foods that can bind to cells in the gut and to blood cells, whereby an inflammatory response is initiated that contributes to problems such as digestive disorders, post-meal fatigue, weight gain and many other challenges to the immune system.

Good health depends on a healthy well-functioning digestive system. Physicians encounter many complaints related to digestion. There could be a variety of reasons for faulty digestion such as food of poor quality and unhealthy eating habits associated with lifestyle. Lectins also contribute to poor digestion that may not be obvious. Even though many people do not feel digestive disturbances, that does not mean lectins are not affecting them.

All plants and animals possess sugar molecules on the surface of each of their cells. These cells play important roles such as in cell communication and protection. But the lectins are not digestible proteins and are capable of selectively binding to these sugars. Each lectin type attaches itself to the surface of a cell to, which it is attracted in our gut and immune system, thereby leaking into our bloodstream. They act like keys to open the doors. Various types of lectins act like different keys and permit those types of lectins to also enter the bloodstream.

Lectins are potent messengers that start and aggravate existing autoimmune diseases such as scleroderma, lupus, rheumatoid arthritis, fibromyalgia, thyroiditis and Irritable Bowel Syndrome (IBS).

Proteins perform many important functions in our bodies. Lectin proteins have the responsibility of helping our red blood cells to reach all of our tissues. While the lectins are in our liver, they help capture and eliminate microorganisms. They are also able to bind to antigens, thereby helping white blood cells to attack and destroy invaders. A good example of this type of lectin is C-reactive protein, which is an important marker of inflammation.

The dark side of lectins is that they cause problems with proteins when they are encountered in the Human body in the form of dietary lectins. While these lectins are in plants, they serve as a type of primitive immune system. When they are consumed, they can cause great problems in our digestive systems, and eventually to the rest of our body.

At this time, animal lectins from ingested meats are not known to be harmful. It is some of the plant lectins that are harmful. The reason for this is that these lectins are almost completely indigestible and not broken down by enzymes. Therefore, dietary lectins from plants remain intact, which enables them to bind to sugars on the surfaces of our blood cells and the lining of our gut. They act as messengers in that area and interrupt proper cell signals and, thereby setting off dangerous inflammatory reactions.

Lectins in our diet damage our delicate intestinal lining and can affect leaky gut and protein digestion. They are also capable of being actively transported across the intestinal membranes and eventually into general circulation where they could attach to other nervous, connective and bladder tissues to cause immune dysfunction and systemic inflammation.

Lectins also contribute to various food sensitivities or food intolerances that provokes the immune system to make antibodies against them. Lectins can cause the type of gut inflammation that has some serious results, which can be sudden and ever lasting. A mild or unnoticeable presence of inflammation in the intestinal tract can take time to build up. It may take years for rheumatoid arthritis or a stubborn weight gain.

Since it is sometimes possible for us to have inflammation without feeling any pain, we can also have the risk of a serious disease or death. One example is the existing cholesterol or fibrin build-up in our veins or arteries are pain free and can cause us to have a stroke or heart attack without warning and can cause death.

Also, at least 6 to 10 years can pass before we are aware of the onset of cancer. This example of a pain free disease is that the onset of cancer in a person's body often does not reveal itself until it is too late. It is very unlikely that a CAT scan or MRI will reveal a cancer the size of the period at the end of this sentence. By that time, the cancer is 6 years old. If the cancer is found to be the size of a small marble, it is then 10 years old. Therefore, the AMAS test could reveal cancer at least 6 to 10 years (with a 95 percent accuracy) before it can establish itself anywhere in our bodies.

The AMAS (Anti Malignan Antibody Serum) test is the only patented and government-approved test that is able to find if our body has a harmful amount of cancer cells, before we experience the onset of full-blown cancer in any part of our body and thereby giving us a much better chance of defeating cancer by early detection and prevention. A much better solution than after-the-fact damage control!

Lectins mimic certain hormones such as insulin and block digestive hormones, which affect our metabolism and can thereby, cause considerable weight gain. This is not an easy counting of calories in or out. Our metabolism is largely controlled by insulin, which in turn affects and is affected by all of our other hormonal influences.

When we are in perfect health, our gastrointestinal tract absorbs food particles for energy consumption by carrying vitamins and minerals across our gut linings and into our bloodstreams. Due to our good metabolism, this produces essential antibodies to protect us from various infections.

If the lining of our intestines becomes agitated long enough, it can become dangerously worn and all of its other crucial functions can be compromised. The most dangerous result of this condition is that our stomach linings and our intestines no longer act as the protective barriers that they are meant to be, in selecting what needs to be kept in and what should be let out. Therefore, gaps form in the walls of our guts, which allow undesired bacteria, undigested food particles, indigestible vegetable lectins, and other toxins cross over and enter into our bloodstreams.

For a long time now, mainstream doctors have not taken seriously what is presently known as "Leaky Gut Syndrome" or Celiac Disease. But, it exists as a real threat with its effects appearing more frequently than the medical profession lets on or even imagines.

When we have a leaky gut, it interrupts normal digestion and prevents our body from obtaining the much needed nutrition required from our food. With this in mind, large food particles have a tendency to enter our bloodstreams and become recognized as foreign pathogens by our immune systems and are therefore attacked. They eventually ignite a widespread systemic inflammation even in our bones and joints.

One common cause is the use of NSAIDS (non-steroidal anti inflammatory drugs) as pain killers along with other medications, which also have a tendency to compromise our digestive systems. Dietary plant lectins are at least equally to blame or possibly more so in many cases.

Natural Killer (NK) cells are a major component of our immune system to fight diseases but the natural killer cell population decreases due to the lectin stimulation in the gut. Lectins have a large impact on the 85 percent of our immune system that lies in our intestinal area and can also stimulate growth in the digestive organs such as the size of the intestines, pancreas and liver.

Some of the symptoms of lectin-related food intolerances are: respiratory problems (asthma, chronic non-infectious coughing), chronic fatigue in general, gastric reflux and stomach upset, hyperactivity, insulin shifts in blood sugar control, easy weight gain and stubborn weight loss, urinary weaknesses with chronic infection, headaches and lack of concentration, water retention and puffiness in the face, under the eyes and extremities, excess mucous and chronic clearing of the throat, joint stiffness and pain (usually) in the morning, abdominal pain and gas with meals,

IBS (irritable bowel syndrome), spastic colon and other intestinal irritation, sinus problems, itchy nose, (hay fever like reactions), congestion and post-nasal drip.

All of the above mentioned symptoms are lectin interactions persisting chronically in some people's diets and which may be reduced by taking a supplemental regimen. Since lectins bind to sugar residues and amino sugars in the gut and on the intestinal cell surfaces, a type of decoy system could be used to sacrifice molecules to bind to lectins and keep them from sticking to our cells and causing damage.

By using decoy sugars when we start a meal, such as with the supplement "Lectin Lock", which allows for the potentially harmful lectins to bind and be eliminated properly by passing all the way through the gut without entering the blood stream.

"Lectin Lock" is a nutritional supplement composed of fucose sugars that are capable of binding to lectins and also microorganisms such as bacteria, yeast and viruses. It also becomes an attachment site for the *Helicobacter pylori* and *Candida albacans* yeast, which is responsible for many ulcers and some forms of gastritis. Lectin Lock prevents their attachment in our GI tract and locks them up to eventually be eliminated from the body. The use of Lectin Lock is a selective therapy that does not upset other balances in the GI tract.

Other studies have shown Lectin Lock has antimicrobial

effects against herpes simplex virus, Human cytomegalo-virus, certain strains of E. coli, all strains tested of *Neisseria meningitides* and Human immunodeficiency virus (HIV).

Research has provided evidence of fucose sugars, which were found to prevent the initial HIV viral attachment to cells necessary for HIV infection. This same concept has been used against malaria through its fucose sugars inhibiting infections and selectively binding to the organisms to prevent them from binding to the cells of the body.

"Lectin Lock" also supports the immune system by engulfing and destroying pathogens by white blood cells and thereby controlling inflammation.

It also helps remove lectins presently in existence and already attached to cells. Better absorption of nutrients is allowed by clearing away the excess mucous resulting from food intolerance or food allergy in the digestive tract and thereby beneficial for malabsorbtion, colitis, ulcers, and other intestinal problems.

The following are Conditions Associated with Leaky Gut Syndrome: Celiac disease, Arthritis, Allergic reactions, Autoimmune disease, Crohn's disease, Inflammatory joint disease (arthritis), Intestinal infections, Environmental illness, Ulcerative colitis, Irritable bowel syndrome, Pancreatic insufficiency, Chronic fatigue syndrome, Liver dysfunction, Psoriasis, Eczema, and Food allergies and sensitivities.

The lectin, WGA (Wheat Germ Agglutin) has been

known to reduce the production of secretin by about 57 percent. Secretin is a digestive hormone responsible for stimulating the pancreas to secrete pancreatic juice. By administering N-acetyl glucosamine, it completely suppressed this effect. N-acetyl glucosamine is the most efficient for bonding to the disruptive wheat lectin, thereby aiding body structure and biological functions such as the immune regulation, inflammation, and signals of cells.

The management of autism is particularly important by suppressing anything that interferes with secretin production. A study of three children with autism and GI (gastrointestinal) problems were given an infusion of secretin and resulted in them being more social and communicative.

Bladerwrack is another lectin-blocking substance and nutritious seaweed component making several contributions. Its fucose sugars bind to lectins and microorganisms such as viruses, bacteria and yeast. It is also a favorite sugar attachment area on the cells surface for the bacteria responsible for ulcers and gastritis (*Helicobacter pylori* and the yeast *Candida albacans*). Therefore, L-fucose is an anti-attachment type of therapy that binds to problem lectins and the two opportunistic pathogens, preventing attachments to them and locking them up to be eliminated from the body.

A supplement of Bladderwrack reduces *H. pylori, C. albacans*, and harmful lectins and, thereby providing selective therapy and does not disrupt other balances of the GI tract. Its antimicrobial effects have also been shown against the herpes simplex virus, Human cytomegalvirus, Human immunodeficiency virus (HIV), certain strains of *E. coli* and all tested strains of *Neisseria meningitides.* Evidence from research and in vitro studies have shown that fucose sugars prevents the initial HIV viral attachment to the cells necessary for HIV infection.

Fucose sugars inhibit the spread of infections by selectively binding to the organisms and to prevent them from binding to the cells of the body. Fucose sugars also support the immune system through engulfing and destroying pathogens by white blood cells and controlling inflammation. Bladderwrack also supports thyroid function to help boost metabolism and help control weight loss.

Okra is the vegetable with a rich lectin-binding protective mucilage to protect the digestive tract from lectins and harmful microorganisms. It also helps remove existing lectins that are already attached to the cells. A combination of okra and the enzyme pepsin could help clear away the excess mucous formed from food intolerance or allergy in the digestive tract, thereby allowing for better absorption of nutrients and help clean the intestine. Okra is beneficial for colitis, ulcers, malabsorption and other intestinal problems.

D-mannose is another common binding sugar and is

capable of binding with lectins in grains and other foods along with microorganisms.

Lectin Lock. 'Lectin Lock' is a new product that claims to be an ideal lectin-locking device and is not a drug. It is composed of all natural ingredients such as Mucins, which are a protein lining our digestive tract as digestive gate-keepers and moistens our saliva and lubricates our food as we eat. The mucins' dense sugar coating, that lectins like to adhere to, resists protein breakdown and maintains mucosal barriers in the gut to protect against food sensitivities of yeast and bacteria.

N-acetyl glucosamine is the most efficient ingredient for bonding to disruptive wheat lectin, thereby aiding body structure and biological functions such as the immune regulation, inflammation and signals of the cells. A very interesting fact is its ability to suppress the anti-secretin effects of the lectin called Wheat Germ Agglutin (WGA).

Research reveals 'Lectin Lock' can be a valuable aid in:

- Reducing inflammation and improving immune function, which lies at the core of chronic disease
- Achieving healthy organs, muscles, and joints
- Repairing the digestive tract and keeping it healthy
- Promoting weight loss through improved metabolism and energy
- Restoring the body's proper water balance

- Promoting healthy detoxification in the liver and the gut
- Helping with any meal in consumption of junk foods or fast foods and highly processed and refined foods that can intensify the effects of dietary lectins

Chapter 6
We Are All Dying of Oxygen Starvation

Thomas Edison was one of the greatest inventors and geniuses of all time who also took an interest in health and disease. He believed in the common sense approach of alternative medicine and could not understand why the medical profession continued treating disease with drugs, when obviously that disease was from a biological imbalance, which drugs cannot correct.

He gave his opinion on these matters by saying, "The doctor of the future will give no medicine but will interest his patients in the care of the Human frame, in diet, and in the cause and prevention of disease." Well, the future that Thomas Edison believed in has just arrived. This is now the time to attempt to stress the importance of treating the cause of all diseases, not merely the symptoms.

Research reveals: About 100 years ago, one of every 150 people had cancer and it has now become one of every three people, and may soon become one of every two during our lifetime. According to the American Cancer Society, 41 percent of Americans probably already have cancer, but they do not know it yet because it has not been detected or diagnosed.

It makes me very sad to think of how many cancer victims die every day, either not knowing about or not trusting amazing cancer alternative treatments. We must educate ourselves and raise our consciousness with accurate information to realize when we are being told the truth and when we are being fed propaganda.

Presently, cancer is the number one killer in America among everyone up to the age of 85. We were one of the healthiest nations on earth 100 years ago but we are not the healthiest nation any more.

Some of the factors contributing to our failing health include:

- The impure water we drink;
- The toxic pesticides that can be found in the fruits and vegetables of the produce sections of our favorite supermarkets;
- The processed food that we eat;

- The toxins in the polluted air we breathe;
- And the limited amount of oxygen in the air that we breathe.

Three essential elements that support life and energy in our body are oxygen, water and nutrients. Oxygen is the most important because we can live several weeks without food, for several days without water, and only a few minutes without oxygen.

Since oxygen is the key to good health, it is the most vital element that is required for Human life. Currently, the Human body is not functioning properly because it is not getting the proper concentrations of oxygen that is currently needed in order to maintain good health.

Oxygen sustains life and controls every function in our body. Our body contains 70 to 100 trillion cells and each of them needs an adequate supply of oxygen to do its job properly. Oxygen and other necessary nutrients are supplied to all of our body's cells, by our circulatory systems, which are composed of at least 75,000 miles of arteries, veins, arterioles, blood vessels, micro vessels, and corpuscles (blood cells).

Oxygen is responsible for cleaning and detoxifying the blood, tissues and it burns off cellular wastes. Oxygen also fights invading microorganisms and soothes our inflammation and pain. If we don't have enough oxygen, our tissues accumulate toxins from metabolic wastes, which may lead to chronic low-grade infections by viruses, bacteria, candida yeasts, or larger parasites, which all give off toxins.

A most dramatic change in the oxygen concentration of our air has taken place within the last 150 to 200 years. Before that time, the oxygen content of our air was about 38% and was accessible for people. This represented the total amount of oxygen in the air at that time. The remaining 62% was composed of other gases such as nitrogen, argon, carbon dioxide, and water vapor.

In reference to a total of anything expressed by way of percentage, that 38% of oxygen in the air represented all of the oxygen in the air of, which 100% was available to people at that time. Assuming that the body has successfully absorbed 100% of the available oxygen needed for its optimum requirement, from the 38% of oxygen in the air at that time, we will now refer to it as the 100% of oxygen in our air at that time. Dividing 100 by 38 gives us a multiplication factor of 2.632.

Presently, there is about 20.9% oxygen concentration in the air we breathe and the remainder of 79.1% is composed of other gases (mostly nitrogen and traces of carbon dioxide, argon, and water vapor). Therefore, we can now calculate the actual amount of our oxygen that is available to us at this time (2.632 x 20. 9) to be 55%.

Also in considering our polluted cities, which with their extra abundance of toxins, pollutants, carbon dioxide, and carbon monoxide, can and do cause the oxygen levels in the air that we breathe, to drop to least to 15%. It now means that we have only 39.48% (2.632 x 15) of preindustrial oxygen levels available to us.

Some of the contributing factors may be the burning of forests, cutting of forests for lumber, the burning of fossil fuels, atmospheric pollution, the depletion of minerals in our soils, and soil erosion. This seriously hinders our efficiency and ability to absorb the optimum levels of oxygen needed to maintain our good health.

Presently, in our polluted cities, oxygen concentrations can be lower than 10% instead of the 38% total oxygen content in the air that people were breathing preindustrially 150 to 200 years ago. There has been a recent report that our atmosphere contains 20% of oxygen, under ideal circumstances. It has also been reported that in many of our polluted cities, the oxygen levels have dropped to 10%.

By using our 2.632 multiplier for the recently reported 20% of oxygen in the air we breathe, the actual oxygen level accessible would be (2.632 x 20) 52.64%. And again, by using our multiplier of 2.632 for that 10% oxygen level in the polluted cities, the actual oxygen levels have dropped (2.632 x 10) to 26.32%. This is a drop of about 73.68% in our oxygen levels and leaves us with only 26.32% of actual oxygen for our accessibility.

The drop in oxygen from our body's optimum oxygen requirement is most detrimental and it causes our body's cells to go haywire, as you will soon realize.

It does not matter where you live; our air is now being saturated with carbon monoxide, thereby saturating the red blood cells of our body and making the hemoglobin unable to carry the much-needed oxygen in order to get enough for the body's metabolism to function properly. This also lowers the amount of oxygen that our bodies are able to absorb.

Many children and adults have blood circulation problems due to blockage that can seriously hinder the oxygen in the blood supply from reaching the body's cells, thereby making us much more susceptible to any and all disease or illness due to the ever decreasing supply of oxygen that is now limited for our bodily functions.

Some people can have between 10 and 85 percent blockage. Even without considering anything else that was previously mentioned about oxygen content of our air, this alone can greatly reduce the oxygen supply to the body anywhere from 10 percent and up at about 85 percent of optimum potential.

If, by some chance, our accessible oxygen level drops and leaves us with only 55% of our optimum oxygen requirement for a period of only 48 hours, we could start getting cancer or any other disease that one can think of.

If our accessible oxygen level drops 40% to leave us with only 60% of our optimum oxygen requirement, all hell seems to break loose, and our cells start going haywire, thereby causing cancer and many other diseases to take hold of us and to ultimately kill us.

Research indicates that the cancers and all other degenerative diseases are caused from oxygen starvation within the body. It does not appear that there is any other way possible to alleviate our reduction of oxygen and increase our body's oxygen supply except by the best, safest, and most affordable way possible, which is through Hydrogen Peroxide and Ozone therapy.

Chapter 7
Hydrogen Peroxide, Ozone, And Oxygen Therapy

First, it is important to briefly explain what ozone is; and why it along with hydrogen peroxide is among the greatest healing miracles of all time.

Most everyone is aware of the ozone layer that surrounds the earth. The ozone layer is an area of the upper atmosphere with a relatively high concentration of ozone that blocks 99 percent of harmful solar ultraviolet radiation.

Since no one knows where the ozone layer begins or ends, no one can accurately measure the altitude of the ozone layer, although "the ozone region" can be estimated to be at an altitude from 6 to 30 miles with its maximum concentration at approximately 15 miles. Ozone is a form of moleculer oxygen, which consists of three atoms of oxygen (O_3) instead of the common two (O_2).

The protective layer of ozone in our atmosphere was formed by an interaction between atmospheric oxygen (O_2) molecules and ultraviolet light from the sun that splits an atmospheric oxygen molecule into two unstable atoms of oxygen.

Since these single atoms of unstable oxygen are very reactive, the single atoms combine to form ozone (O_3), which is composed of three atoms of oxygen (O_3). Ozone molecules are very unstable and quickly give up extra atoms of oxygen to falling rainwater, thereby forming hydrogen peroxide (H_2O_2).

Hydrogen Peroxide is somewhat like a molecule of water with an extra atom of oxygen attached to it. H_2O_2 occurs throughout nature and is produced by every cell in our body. When the extra oxygen atom (O) is released from hydrogen peroxide (H_2O_2), it is very biochemically reactive and is referred to as a free radical. During the past several years, it was believed that these free radicals were responsible for all types of our ailments and even premature aging.

Dr. Denham Harmon developed the free-radical theory of aging in the 1950's. He reported that free radicals are molecules that have a chemically active oxygen atom attached to them and, thereby caused damage to cells and lead to both aging and cancer.

From the beginning, it seemed that extra oxygen was always damaging and antioxidants were good by being responsible for anti-aging protection. But our bodies create and use free radicals to destroy harmful bacteria, viruses, and fungi. The cells that are responsible for fighting infection and foreign invaders in the body (our white blood cells) make hydrogen peroxide and use it to oxidize any of the offending foreign invaders.

Presently, it does not appear that all free-radical reactions are bad. For example, oxygen helps cleansing enzymes to remove toxins, and used by the immune system to attack invading bacteria, stimulates natural killer (NK) cells to attack cancer cells as they attempt to spread throughout the body. Our cells have the ability to produce hydrogen peroxide, which is essential for life. It is now known to be a basic requirement for good health and is not some undesirable by-product or toxin.

Dr. Charles Farr found that intravenous hydrogen peroxide administration stimulated oxidative enzymes in the body to help cleanse out toxins. This almost doubled the enzyme's metabolic rate, which may partially account for the benefits observed.

One might wonder how something that produces free radicals can possibly have a therapeutic effect. Well, the damage from free radicals is from the chronic exposure due to free-radical oxygen (part of more complex molecules). The stimulation of the oxidative enzymes and the process of oxygenation may account for the positive effects observed of hydrogen peroxide.

There was a time when rains carried ozone, along with hydrogen peroxide, and nourished the world's vegetation, which was a big help to agriculturalists and farmers. Since the air is loaded with pollutants, toxins, and other unhealthy components, much of the available ozone is unstable and very reactive; thereby it is depleted from the atmosphere by reacting with the air pollutants while purifying the air. Because of its depletion from natural rainwater, farmers now spray their crops with diluted forms of hydrogen peroxide to help ensure optimal plant growth.

The ozone layer is essential for Human life because it absorbs much of the Sun's harmful ultraviolet radiation, thereby preventing this radiation from entering living cells and destroying the deoxyribonucleic acid (DNA) of many life forms on our planet. If the ozone layer ceased to exist, high concentrations of ultraviolet light radiation would bombard the earth, thereby inducing cancer to break out in all living things and would eventually cause all forms of life, as we know it, to become extinct.

Ozone Layer damage each year is attributed to:
    Volcanic Eruptions 1 to 5 percent
    Natural Resources 15 to 20 percent
    Human Activity 75 to 85 percent

The Human body is currently getting much lower concentrations of oxygen than it actually needs for proper functioning. The total content of dissolved oxygen in our blood and in our cells is less than the needed amount for good health, proper metabolism, and high energy. Because of this, the body has developed greater susceptibility to chronic diseases when its optimum oxygen levels are decreased. Since oxygen is the most vital nutrient for our bodies, our internal organs become diseased and they age much faster, whenever our body's necessary levels of oxygen are reduced.

As we age, our immune systems become much weaker and this in turn, threatens our health by permitting unwanted organisms and pathogens to breed and to spread. Research indicates that when oxygen is withdrawn from healthy cells they can more easily turn into cancer cells.

Our bodies must maintain an aerobic environment, in the sense that we need plenty of oxygen for our cells to perform their basic metabolic functions (respiration, growth, repair, and reproduction) by burning glucose. If our cells become surrounded with wastes, oxygen cannot reach them, thereby preventing our cells from functioning properly. When this happens, oxygen no longer reaches the cells; and the environment in the body becomes "anaerobic" (without oxygen); and negative changes begin to happen.

Cells become diseased and then can actually prefer to

live and multiply in an oxygen poor or anaerobic environment, and thereby increase in quantity in an environment filled with wastes. This negative environment is perfect for initiating and sustaining cancer. Therefore, an increase in oxygen in our bodies can only benefit us by assuring normal cellular functioning and preventing cancer and other diseases.

Hydrogen Peroxide Therapy and Ozone Therapy are powerful tools for curing all diseases and for the prevention of all cancers. Hundreds of diseases are symptoms of the underlying cause, which was proven by the three-time-nominated and two-time Noble Prize winning German scientist, Otto Warburg. Since 1926, Warburg proved and made it known that when a cell is deprived of about 40 percent of its normal requirement of oxygen, its respiration is irreversibly damaged.

The resulting damage causes the cell to begin to ferment sugar anaerobically (without oxygen) producing carbon monoxide and lactic acid, and at only 1/6 of the energy of normal cellular aerobic oxidation. The cell eventually loses its control on growth and begins to grow uncontrollably... which is by definition what we call "cancer". Therefore, it is necessary to supply oxygen at the cellular level to be able to destroy cancer and especially to prevent it in the first place.

Oxygen starvation at the cellular level eventually causes more degenerative diseases such as: AIDS, Acne,

Allergies, Altitude sickness, Alzheimer's Disease, Angina, Arrhythmia, Arteriosclerosis, Arthritis, Asthma, Bacterial Infections, Bronchitis, Burns, Cancer, Candidiasis, Cardiovascular Disease, Cerebral Vascular Disease, High Cholesterol, Chronic Pain, Cirrhosis of the liver, Cluster Headaches, Colitis, C. O. P. D. (Chronic Obstructive Pulmonary Disease), Cystitis, Diabetes Type II, Diabetic Gangrene, Diabetic Retinopathy, Digestion Problems, Eczema, Epstein-Barr Infection, Fungus, Gangrene, Gingivitis, Gum Disease, Headaches, Hepatitis, Herpes, Herpes Simplex, Herpes Zoster, HIV Infection, Influenza, Insect Bites, Leg Ulcers, Leukemia, Lupus Erythematosis, Lymphoma, Metastatic Carcinoma, Migraine Headaches, Mononucleosis, Multiple Sclerosis, Open sores and wounds, Parasitic infections, Periodontal Disease, Proctitis, Prostatitis, Rheumatoid Arthritis, Shingles, Sinusitis, Sore Throat, Temporal Arthritis, Trichomoniasis, Ulcers, Vascular Diseases, Vascular headaches, Viral Infections, more unmentioned diseases (some of which are 30 new diseases discovered in the last 20 years), and probably countless other diseases not even discovered yet.

Research also indicates that all diseases are anaerobic and cannot survive in an oxygen rich environment. Therefore, all diseases are symptoms of the same underlying cause, which is attributed to the body's lack of oxygen or oxygen starvation.

Our cells normally function by burning sugar (glucose)

in the presence of oxygen to provide energy, which results in the waste products carbon dioxide and water. If insufficient oxygen is present at the cellular level, the burn will be incomplete, which causes the formation of carbon monoxide and lactic acid. The body cannot easily get rid of carbon monoxide (CO) and its presence prevents hemoglobin (in our blood cells) from picking up fresh oxygen.

This leads to hypothermia (low body temperature). Hypothermia is followed by lactic acid build-up in the body, clogging the nerve pathways and eventually calcifying them and causing degeneration and ultimately death.

Much-needed oxygen is unavailable to oxidize these built up toxins; they continue to build up. The blood carries a heavy load of sludge and toxins that get deposited in our fat cells. The fluid composition of the body continues to get dirtier, overtaxing our kidneys and liver and lymphatic systems, and results in a variety of diseases and eventually death.

If Hydrogen Peroxide Therapy or Ozone Therapy is started, it causes an immediate increase in red blood cell numbers, which leads to an increase in the amount of oxygen carried to and released in our tissues. This in turn causes stimulation for the production of a whole host of essential enzymes, which then act as free radical scavengers and cell protectors.

Oxygen deficiency can be caused by many and various factors such as toxins reaching our cells and blocking their supply of oxygen. All carcinogens hinder necessary and normal cellular respiration. I believe it is a waste of time and money to search for more carcinogenic substances because they tend to obscure the real cause of cancer.

Since the cause of cancer is largely misunderstood, its proper treatment is misunderstood and is not properly undertaken. Cancer is entirely preventable and treatable as it is actually caused by oxygen starvation of our cells. Reversing this oxygen-starvation by increasing oxygen flow in our blood and to our cells by any and all means available IS the one and only genuine cure for cancer.

In order to destroy cancer, massive amounts of oxygen are required at the cellular level. Ozone has been used with great success for over 75 years. Ozone should be taken in as many different ways as possible, to flood the cells with oxygen. A direct injection into the tumor is possible for treatment of breast cancer. For people with liver cancer, an injection into the portal vein is necessary, as developed by Dr. William Turska. Other treatments are usually done with intravenous placed into the arm.

Ozone also has the ability to prevent cancer if sufficient oxygen is provided to the cells and not allowing concentrations to drop below 60 percent of normal oxygen concentration requirements. Ozone generators are currently being used by many people to keep their cellular oxygen levels high in order to prevent disease.

If we want to eliminate toxins from our bodies every day and keep our cells supplied with their required amounts of oxygen, thereby preventing our cells from switching from aerobic (oxygen-rich) to anaerobic (without oxygen), then taking ozone on a daily basis should be a small price for each of us to pay.

There is much being said about cholesterol and clogging of the arteries. But the intake of cholesterol is not directly related to cholesterol levels. Apparently, the problem is caused by chlorine reacting with the cholesterol and causing it to coagulate onto the walls of the arteries and causing plaque build-up. The major sources of chlorine are the drinking water supply and the salt (sodium chloride) in our food. Chlorine appears to be the main culprit for both heart disease and for high blood pressure.

By ingesting ozone over a period of time, it scours out the arteries by oxidizing the plaque and, thereby cleaning the circulatory system to allow blood to flow properly. Ozone is also very helpful in reducing the clumping of red blood cells and enables them to pick up oxygen in the lungs, which is crucial to microcirculation through our fine capillaries.

Again, Cancer is entirely preventable and treatable as it is actually caused by oxygen starvation of the cell. Reversing this oxygen-starvation by increasing oxygen flow in our blood and to our cells by any and all means available IS the one and only genuine cure for cancer. Ozone and Hydrogen Peroxide bio-oxidative therapies are the best ways to accomplish this.

Chapter 8
The Cause of Cancer Was Discovered by Dr. Otto Warburg

Oxygen is the most vital element required for Human life and the key to good health. Insufficient oxygen and disease has been firmly established. Dr. Otto Warburg was awarded the Noble Prize in 1931 and in 1944 for discovering the cause of cancer. He said, "Cancer has only one prime cause. The prime cause of cancer is the replacement of normal oxygen respiration of body cells by an anaerobic (oxygen-less) cell respiration."

Our cells function by burning sugar (glucose) in oxygen to provide energy and results in the waste products of carbon dioxide and water. If insufficient oxygen is present at the cellular level, the burn will be incomplete, thereby causing the fermentation of carbon monoxide and lactic acid.

Since the body cannot easily get rid of carbon monoxide, which prevents hemoglobin (in our blood) from picking up fresh oxygen, the body temperature is lowered and is followed by a lactic acid buildup in the body, clogging the nerve pathways and eventually calcifying and causing degeneration.

Since 1926 and due to the work of Dr. Otto Warburg, it was known that as soon as the available oxygen to a cell drops below 60 percent of the cell's normal requirement, its respiration is irreversibly damaged. The cell tends to go haywire and become anaerobic. Upon this happening, the cell is forcibly switched from oxidation for energy production to fermentation, which is an inferior method of energy production. This cell can never return to its former state of oxygen respiration. Therefore, this cell reproduces copies of itself wildly. This is the condition known as cancer.

Dr. Warburg made it known that if any substance deprives a cell of oxygen it is a carcinogen, if the affected cell is not killed. In 1966, Dr. Warburg mentioned that it was useless to search for new carcinogens due to the same result of each one being the same with their reaction of depriving cellular oxygen. The search for new carcinogens obscured the prime cause of cancer, which was the lack of cellular oxygen.

In 1929, a book named *Ozone and Its Therapeutic*

Action was published in the United States by authors who were also the leading heads of American hospitals. It listed 114 diseases and their treatment with ozone therapy.

In 1933, a Dr. Simmons, who set out to destroy all medical treatments that were competitive to the drug industry, headed the American Medical Association. The suppression of ozone therapy started then and it continues in the United States to this very day.

In 1952, The National Cancer Institute endorsed Dr. Warburg's findings that the lack of oxygen plays the major role in causing cells to become cancerous. Dr. Harry Goldblatt continued the research, published his findings in *The Journal of Experimental Medicine* in 1953, and confirmed that the lack of oxygen plays the major role in causing cells to become cancerous.

Chapter 9
Physicians Recommending the Use of Oxygen Therapy

Dr. Albert Wahl said, "Disease is due to deficiency in the oxidation process of the body, leading to an accumulation of toxins. These toxins are ordinarily burned in normal oxidation."

Dr. Wendell Hendricks of the Hendricks Research Foundation wrote: "Cancer is a condition within the body where the oxidation has become so depleted that the body cells have degenerated beyond control. The body is so overloaded with toxins that it sets up a tumor mass to harbor these poisons and remove them from general activity within the body."

He further states," The true cause of allergy is a lowered

oxidation process within the body, causing the body to be sensitive to substances entering. Only when the oxidative mechanism is restored to a higher state of efficiency can the sensitivity be eliminated."

In 1985, Dr. Stephen Levine stated, "Hypoxia, or the lack of oxygen in the tissues, is the fundamental cause of all degenerative disease."

Dr. Norman McVea stated in 1985, "When the body has ample oxygen, it produces enough energy to optimize metabolism and eliminate accumulated toxic wastes in the tissues. Natural immunity is achieved when the immune system is not burdened with heavy "toxic buildup." Detoxification occurs when oxygen is introduced into the system."

Dr. Christiaan N. Barnard (1922-2001) was a South African surgeon who was world famous for performing the first Human-to-Human being heart transplant in 1967.

In March of 1987, Dr. Barnard stated emphatically, "Yes, I use Hydrogen Peroxide Therapy every day to ward off diseases that come with age and to help with my arthritis." He later recanted this declaration due to pressure from the big pharmaceutical companies and the AMA, but he never stopped using his oxygen therapy program. It was also rumored that he has dated Gina Lollabrigida and Sophia Loren. It appears The Oxygen Therapy Program seemed to be working very well and appeared to restore some of his youthful energy and libido.

In the *Journal of the American Association of Physicians*, Dr. W. Spencer Way stated, "Insufficient oxygen means insufficient biological energy that can result in anything from mild fatigue to life threatening disease. The link between insufficient oxygen and disease has now been firmly established. The more oxygen we have in our system, the more energy we produce."

In *Oxygen Therapies: A New Way of Approaching Disease*, Dr. Ed McCabe stated, "The large majority of those infectious microbes that cause us so much illness and pain are ANAEROBIC... A big word that means they live and proliferate best in environments where there is LITTLE OR NO OXYGEN."

In the *Journal of Experimental Medicine*, Dr. Harry Goldblatt stated, "Lack of oxygen clearly plays a major role in causing cells to become cancerous."

The winner of the Noble Prize for Cancer Research, Otto Warburg stated, "Cancer has only one prime cause. It is the replacement of normal oxygen respiration of the body's cells by an anaerobic (i.e. oxygen deficient) cell respiration."

Dr. Arthur Guyton, M. D. stated, "All chronic suffering is caused from a lack of oxygen at the cell level."

Dr. Parris Kidd, Ph.D. Stated, "We can look at oxygen deficiency as the single greatest cause of all disease."

In the August 22, 1980 edition of journal *SCIENCE* (Vol. 209), there was a report written by Dr. Michael

Carpendale entitled: Ozone Selectively Inhibits Growth of Cancer Cells."

On February 17-19, 1989, the First International Conference of Bio-oxidative Medicine was held in Dallas/Ft. Worth, Texas, during which various physicians presented papers on the infusion of hydrogen peroxide therapy. Since that time, this non-profit foundation has attracted many physicians who also presented much of their work with patients.

Dr. William Campbell Douglas, M. D. believes the Baylor University Medical Center may "have gone a long way toward proving that H_2O_2 (hydrogen peroxide) dripped into the leg and carotid vessels of patients known to have arteriosclerosis will clear those arteries of disease.

An extremely useful treatment of Chelation Therapy cannot clean the hardened plaque out of large heart arteries. Research has revealed that diluted hydrogen peroxide accomplished the separation of lipids from the arterial wall, more than 20 years ago. Dr. Douglas also related that "the investigators also reported the improvement is not temporary."

Chapter 10
Ozone and Hydrogen Peroxide Therapy

Ozone and Hydrogen Peroxide therapy may be the closest thing to a miraculous cure-all for Human disorders that any of us will ever encounter. This therapy has been deliberately suppressed by the FDA (Food and Drug Administration) and the AMA (American Medical Association), who actually care more about their own financial interests than helping people to stay healthy.

This could easily make any one of us angry because we have all had friends or relatives who have suffered needlessly or died from preventable diseases because this information was not available to them. And even worse, this lifesaving information has been deliberately withheld... all for financial profit!

At the present time, there are confusing practices for treating diseases of every part of the Human body. The average person cannot understand that medicines are complicated within specialized fields of cardiology, dermatology, endocrinology, gynecology, neurology, ophthalmology, urology, oncology (for cancer), gerontology (old age diseases), and with each of them having their own unique and particular methods of treatment. This is not a clever appeal to make you fearful and cause you to make any decisions before you first investigate their validity.

The field of medicine has various theories for the cause of diseases and how to eliminate them from the Human body. Our trillion dollar medical and pharmaceutical industries are the largest in the world and yet we have a larger percentage of sick people in the United States than any other place in the world.

Even though superficially the medical profession has honorable intentions of helping people and healing us of disease, it has been very ineffective by preferably favoring expensive profit motivated procedures, selling drugs, and convincing us to accept unproven, ineffective, and experimental at best treatments and procedures. Most of them only relieve the symptoms or the pain of our diseases if we are "lucky". Practically all drugs that are used have horrible side effects, which by far outnumber their benefits, and that may create even more problems for our health.

Oxygen is responsible for 90 percent of all biological

energy metabolism within our bodies. While we are breathing, the absorbed oxygen enters the bloodstream and is delivered to our cells and body tissues. This process raises tissue oxygen levels to enable healthy cells to survive and multiply more rapidly and to create a stronger immune system.

The bio-oxidative therapy of Ozone and Hydrogen Peroxide stimulates the movement of oxygen atoms from the bloodstream to the cells more than usual and causes an increase in oxygen levels. The higher levels of oxygen in the tissues cause apoptosis (suicide) to take place among the bad bacteria and viruses because they are anaerobic and cannot survive in an oxygen rich environment.

Germs, bacteria, viruses, protozoa, and other pathogens do not cause disease; but they do seek the environments where they can survive well... especially in oxygen-deprived bodies.

Ozone and hydrogen peroxide are the easiest substances available that can effectively oxygenate the body by giving up their oxygen atoms, and produce an oxygen rich environment in the body. Hydrogen peroxide is more readily available and easy to use. The FDA (Food and Drug Administration) has given hydrogen peroxide the GRAS designation (Generally Recognized as Safe).

Hydrogen peroxide creates an oxygen rich environment in the body that virtually cures you of all diseases caused by viruses, toxins, parasites, yeast, disease microorganisms, harmful bacteria, protozoa, and other pathogens, while contributing to the vitality for good healthy cells. Hydrogen peroxide (food grade) therapy provides the most abundant and essential element of the Human body.

Of all the different elements and nutrients that your body needs, only oxygen is in very critical demand and an insufficient supply makes the body develop diseases because diseases thrive in an oxygen poor environment.

Profiteering of any kind is NOT the motive for the information contained in this chapter regarding therapeutic benefits of food grade H_2O_2 (neither is it the motive for this book nor for ANY of the information contained herein).

Food grade H_2O_2 is a chemical that has a very low profit margin, thereby making it very unlikely to be overpriced by profiteers. It is easily available and costs an average of less than 10 cents per day for the recommended dosage, which takes less than one minute to administer. Since hydrogen peroxide therapy goes back 170 years and because it is still being used today, it was able to withstand the test of time.

Oxygen has never been given credit as the cure for virtually all diseases because it was seldom used by the medical profession for curing or preventing diseases. Science and medicine always knew that oxygen is the most vital element that supports life. Research reveals that the primary cause of all diseases is linked to oxygen deficiency.

You can oxygenate your body with food grade H_2O_2,

with a relatively simple procedure without the aid of a doctor and duplicate healing results in your own home in a minute or less, three times a day. By using this therapy, it will allow you to control your health and heal yourself of virtually all diseases.

Hydrogen peroxide therapy oxygenates your body and enables it to have an oxygen rich environment, thereby making it uninhabitable by harmful viruses, toxins, disease microorganisms, harmful bacteria, parasites, yeast protozoa and other pathogens. This eventually enables your body to heal itself.

It has been proven that hydrogen peroxide and ozone has been used to treat just about every type of illness. Disease-causing viruses, cancer cells, arthritis microbes, colds, and flu are all anaerobic organisms and cells in that, like most primitive lower forms of life, they use sugar in the absence of oxygen to survive.

Hydrogen Peroxide is produced by almost every cell in the Human body for many different reasons. It plays some very important roles in the body's immune system to destroy foreign substances and toxins to our body.

Our immune system also helps produce hydrogen peroxide as a first line of defense against viruses, harmful bacteria, toxins, disease microorganisms, parasites, protozoa, yeast, viruses, and fungi. Therefore, it is currently being used by doctors all over the world as an oxidative therapy to treat various diseases. It is also being used on many patients who suffer with chronic conditions that have not responded to conventional medical treatments.

Among the group of doctors who have used hydrogen peroxide therapy was the late Charles H. Farr, MD, Ph.D., who was nominated for the Nobel Prize in Medicine, during the year of 1933, for his work as pioneer in oxidative research. He claimed to have discovered "a positive metabolic effect to intravenous infusions of hydrogen peroxide." Dr. Farr was a founder of the "American College for Advancement in Medicine" (ACAM), the founding father and director of the International Bio-Oxidative Medical Foundation (IBOMF), and its close affiliate, the International Oxidative Medical Association (IOMA).

Dr. Farr summarized the therapeutic potential of hydrogen peroxide therapy in simple terms by stating, "No distinct group of patients or classifications of disease at this time can be considered the proper selections." Since intravenous infusions of hydrogen peroxide provide oxygenation to highly toxic tissue, kill or inhibit certain bacteria, yeast, viruses, protozoa and parasites, and, since it has a stimulatory effect on the immune system, many different pathological conditions seem to respond to intravenous hydrogen peroxide therapy."

Hydrogen peroxide and ozone therapy is based on the knowledge that the accumulated toxins in the body are normally burned during the oxidation process, whereby the substance is changed from the effect of unstable oxygen's reaction on it. The oxidation process breaks down the toxins into carbon dioxide and water and, thereby eliminating them from the body. When your body's oxygen system is deficient and cannot eliminate them, you can incur a toxic reaction, which can result in deadly diseases if you have a chronic problem with poor oxygenation.

Dr. Douglas reported that "Dr. Edward C. Rosenow, author of 450 published medical papers and associate at the Mayo Clinic for over 60 years proved [more than] 90 years ago (in 1914) that bacteria could be found consistently in the lymph nodes that drain joints (*Journal of the American Medical Association*, April 11, 1914). He was probably the first scientist to postulate that H_2O_2 would help arthritis because of its ability to supply oxygen to oxygen-hating organisms causing arthritis. (*Streptococcus viridans*)".

Hydrogen peroxide is involved in various metabolic pathways such as carbohydrate, protein, and fat metabolism, along with vitamin and mineral metabolism, or any other system that you may wish to explore. Intravenous infusion of H_2O_2 (hydrogen peroxide) demonstrates its metabolic effects by its ability to oxidize almost any physiological or pathological substance and has proved to have therapeutic value.

The two ways to administer pure "food grade" hydrogen peroxide for medical purposes consists of IV (intravenous) or orally. Some clinics have been successfully treating patients with both.

Pure "food grade" hydrogen peroxide is an uncontaminated substance and does not contain anything harmful or toxic. It has been known for decades that it forms powerful protections of cellular and metabolic strength by joining with other elements in our body to make it an extremely powerful biocide, anti-fungal and virus killer.

Research reveals the use of H_2O_2, by either infusion or orally, stimulates the oxidative enzymes and is more important than the amount of oxygen it supplies. Just because there are a number of commercial products that may contain more oxygen than hydrogen peroxide, that does not mean that they would have more biological activity. The big difference lies in the terminology of Oxygenation and Oxidation when it is applied to biochemical reactions of which I will give a brief explanation.

Hydrogen peroxide is an effective oxygenator and a powerful oxidizer. There is an apparent difference between Oxygenation (caused by oxygenators) and Oxidation (caused by oxidizers). Oxygenation increases the use of oxygen at the cellular level, increases the oxygen content in the blood, and improves both cellular oxygen uptake and utilization by the cells.

Oxygen serves as the final proton (H+... Hydrogen ion) acceptor in most of our metabolic pathways. When molecular oxygen combines with these acidic hydrogen ions, water is formed. That is why we sweat, exhale, and urinate a lot of water. Most biomolecules are formed by dehydration ("water out") synthesis. Conversely we need to maintain good hydration because water is necessary to metabolize biomolecules by hydrolysis ("water splitting") into smaller molecules.

Two of these processes, for example, are the building up of proteins from amino acids by splitting out water molecules or the breakdown of polysaccharides (sugar chains such as starches) by inserting water (H+ and OH-) to yield simple sugars. Again, Oxygen serves as the acceptor for free-radical Hydrogen Ions in our bodies.

Oxidation refers to the process of transferring electrons between two or more molecules. Hydrogen Peroxide is an oxidizer and is essential within the body for the processes of life. Therefore, H_2O_2 is of therapeutic use as part of Bio-oxidative Medicine.

Research has shown that oral or intravenous hydrogen peroxide and ozone therapy have been used to treat just about every type of disease by killing bacteria, viruses, fungi, parasites, yeast, etc.

Special types of white blood cells (lymphocytes and phagocytes) in our immune system naturally produce hydrogen peroxide as the first line of defense against parasites, toxins, bacteria, protozoa, viruses and yeast. If we could help provide some extra hydrogen peroxide for the body to use, it would offer additional support by enhancing our immune system.

The very simple molecule of hydrogen peroxide is

produced by almost every cell in the body and plays a very important role in oxidative metabolism. Many people in the world may believe biological oxidation to be harmful because it may produce free radicals, which can cause lipid peroxidation and membrane damage. Therefore, many anti-oxidant products are being promoted to prevent it. Some researchers feel peroxidation has a useful purpose in biochemical balance.

Hydrogen peroxide is an oxidizer of, which its principle reaction is to accept electrons in reduction/oxidation reactions of the body for, which it has nothing to do with "oxygen" or "Oxygenation." Hydrogen Peroxide increases the rate of oxidation in the body because it stimulates oxidative enzymes and not because it produces oxygen.

The purpose of the hydrogen peroxide molecule is that it functions in the body as a hormonal messenger, aids membrane support, regulates body heat, improves immune function and other important metabolic functions. The body purposely uses hydrogen peroxide to produce the Hydroxyl Radicals to kill viruses, yeasts, fungi, protozoa, bacteria, and parasites, which is not attributed to increasing the amount of available oxygen. Since hydrogen peroxide is an oxidizer, it is involved in the oxidative process of removing an electron from molecules and thereby changing electrical energy of the molecule into an oxidized state.

The general public, as well as many practicing physicians,

are unaware that hydrogen peroxide therapy has been used for over one hundred years. Presently, many clinics in the United States and Mexico are using hydrogen peroxide therapy on a routine basis and it is usually given by IV (intravenous injection).

Our immune system's very first lines of defense against all microorganism invaders are our white blood cells, which bring into play, the lymphocytes, phagocytes, and macrophages (as garbage disposals cells), which use hydrogen peroxide to oxidize these foreign invaders, which consist of parasites, toxins, bacteria, protozoa, viruses, bacteria, viruses and yeast. Vitamin "C" plays a very effective role in this process by promoting the hydrogen peroxide use against these same foreign invaders.

Since all body tissues contain catalase (an enzyme in the blood and tissue) and when Hydrogen peroxide is in the presence of catalase it is reduced to oxygen and water. Therefore, there is a strong belief that added hydrogen peroxide may be effective and safe against certain organisms that thrive in an oxygen poor environment.

Some physicians discovered use of hydrogen peroxide therapy effective against various types of cancer, leukemia, arterial circulation problems, coronary heart disease, colitis, gum disease, various children's diseases, arthritis and many more. Since the early nineteenth century, hydrogen peroxide therapy was successfully used in medicine for many bacterial diseases when no other treatment was effective.

The ability of hydrogen peroxide to kill bacteria in the Human body has been described in a medical textbook back in 1922. Dr. Edward Rosenow (1875-1966) was a physician and research scientist with the Mayo Clinic for over 40 years. He found the causes of over 35 diseases and authored 450 medical reports.

Dr. Rosenow basically believed that our body is like a world with millions of microorganisms (little creatures searching for their own habitat, food and environment). They can be compared to animals living in different climates of our world, whereby they eat different foods, multiply, prey upon others, infect, and pollute environment.

As these little microorganisms invade our bodies and seek out their proper habitats, they are responsible for:

- causing inflammatory arthritis by chewing away at joints
- cementing bones together with calcium waste
- forming stones in the liver and kidneys, due to their bite
- leaving hard deposits on the walls of our arteries by living in our arteries
- short-circuiting some of the electronics in the central computer of the brain by clinging to the lining of the nervous system
- attacking and entering our cells, thereby causing the cell to lose its specific function.

Dr. Rosenow developed a method by which microorganisms in the body could be eliminated or controlled with hydrogen peroxide therapy. He discovered that hydrogen peroxide was a safe effective antimicrobial and antiviral agent that he spent many years to find. He died in 1966 without seeing his discovery generally accepted.

Dr. Edward Rosenow's friend, Father Wilhelm, who was a Catholic priest and chemistry teacher, committed himself to publicize the miraculous benefits of hydrogen peroxide.

During the 1970's, Father Wilhelm presented Dr. Rosenow's research to many large pharmaceutical companies and was unsuccessful. Even though Dr. Rosenow's work with hydrogen peroxide was very interesting and important, it appeared that Father Wilhelm received the same disappointing response because hydrogen peroxide was a natural and inexpensive substance that could not be patented therefore, it had no commercial value.

Dr. Hans Alfred Nieper of Hanover, Germany was a well-known German orthomolecular physician and an oncologist known to be treating Cancer patients with Ozone and Hydrogen Peroxide and was consulted by comedian Red Buttons, actor Yul Brynner and our former President Ronald Regan. After President Ronald Regan went to Germany for his cancer treatment, he came back cured and lived another 17 years before he finally died of something else.

Dr Nieper was born in Germany in 1928. In Germany, he was the founder and the first 5-year president of the German Society of Oncology. This biologically oriented cancer society grew tremendously and is now the biggest cancer society in all of Europe. He was also a life member of the German Society of Natural Scientists and Physicians.

Dr. Hans A. Nieper arrived at Memorial Sloan-Kettering Cancer Center (MSKCC) in New York in June 1974. President Nixon declared "War on Cancer" in December 1971, which created an atmosphere of excitement. Soon after his arrival, Dr. Nieper discovered there was another side in the "War on Cancer" that few people at MSKCC knew, and was the highly controversial alternative type of treatment that already existed in Germany, Mexico, and underground in the United States itself. The Public Affairs Office cautioned patients away from such non-conventional approaches.

Dr. Nieper was astounded by the fact that controversial alternative type of treatments were quietly and sympathetically being explored in private meetings on the 13th floor of Sloan-Kettering's Howard Building where scientific leaders Robert A. Good, MD, PhD, Lloyd Old, MD and Lewis Thomas MD had their headquarters to pioneer the immunological approach to cancer. Dr. Nieper was the youthful and obviously brilliant German doctor that was consulted the most. One of the scientific leaders sent his own mother to be treated with beneficial results obtained by Dr. Nieper.

There were complaints that Dr. Nieper swayed the leaders of Sloan-Kettering, Drs. Good, Old, and Thomas. Although they were world-famous immunologists, they did not have much experience in the application of non-conventional concepts to cancer patients. Therefore, they became pupils of Dr. Nieper, so to speak. Dr. Nieper is also world famous for his treatment of multiple sclerosis with hydrogen peroxide therapy.

In the USA, Dr. Nieper was an active member of the New York Academy of Sciences, The American Association for the Advancement of Sciences, The American College of Nutrition and other societies. He has passed away in his sleep on October 21, 1998 and left behind a wealth of information that will be beneficial for generations to come.

During an interview by NHF videographer Jeff Harsh, Dr. Hans Nieper, the ozone treatment doctor, talked about his work with colon cancer. Although he said he could not divulge the name of his patients he said; "President Regan is a very nice man." He also said "You wouldn't believe how many FDA officials or relatives or acquaintances of FDA officials come to see me as patients in Hanover. You wouldn't believe this, or directors of the American Medical Association (AMA), or American Cancer Association, or the presidents of orthodox cancer institutes. That's the fact."

This appears to be a very odd fact that these VIP's had enough money and sought to have this treatment of ozone therapy in Germany because it was good enough for them, but it wasn't allowed for the common people in our own country.

With 35 percent of "food grade" being diluted by using suggested measured quantities of drops in distilled water. The dosages and number of oral treatments are increased daily over a number of weeks.

Many researchers and reputable physicians have made legitimate claims of safety and efficacy of using hydrogen peroxide therapy. If we can insure that our bodies are sufficiently oxygenated, we can eliminate toxins and cure disease.

In scientific studies, Hydrogen Peroxide (Food Grade) and Medical Ozone, when properly introduced into the body in repeated applications, removes accumulated toxins, inactivates viruses, bacteria, fungi, yeast, protozoa, parasites and carcinomas in disease cells. All of these are anaerobic and cannot survive in an oxygen-rich environment.

Ozone therapy was found to be an extremely safe medical therapy free from side effects. The German Medical Society for Ozone Therapy performed a study in 1980 and polled 644 of their therapists regarding their 384,775 patients, which totaled 5,579,238 administered ozone treatments.

Only 40 cases of side effects were noted and represented a very low rate of .000007 percent with only four fatalities. This essentially proves Ozone Therapy is the safest medical therapy that was ever devised. Over 8,000 doctors in Germany use Ozone therapy daily.

Medical Ozone therapy has been recognized in 16 nations, which include the following: Bulgaria, Cuba, Czech Republic, France, Germany, Israel, Mexico, Romania, and Russia. Access - type bills, to ensure that alternative therapies are available to consumers, has been passed for eleven additional states in the United States, which are: AK, CO, GA, MN, NY, NC, OH, OK, OR, SC, and WA. Efforts to pass similar legislation are also underway in CA, DE, FL, KY, MA, MO, VA, and WY.

Once Hydrogen Peroxide or Ozone Therapy is started, it eliminates toxicity of the body by cleaning all of the body fluids by killing bacteria, parasites, yeast, protozoa, fungus, inhibiting viruses and oxidizing immune complexes.

Again, I must remind you that the following information as well as the rest of the information in this book, is for educational purposes only. It is not to be considered diagnostic or prescriptive advice. Please see your doctor for medical advice and further references. See your doctor.

Before you use hydrogen peroxide on your own, it is advisable to research it, because a few basic errors that you make can cause problems. If you have doubt as to the use of oral hydrogen peroxide and its use as IV (intravenous) treatment, make your own judgment by a study of the issues. Then find a physician who has experience and knows what he/she is doing.

Food grade hydrogen peroxide comes in 12%, 17% or 35% solutions. Using distilled water, it must be diluted to a minimum 3.5% solution before it can be used for therapeutic purposes. If any concentration of hydrogen peroxide is above 10%, it can cause neurological damage.

If hydrogen peroxide is accidently spilled on yourself, you will feel a temporary stinging sensation with a lightening of skin color. You should quickly rinse that area thoroughly under running water. Your skin color will return in 30 minutes and possibly up to one hour. No toxins have been absorbed and no permanent skin damage has been done. If it accidently gets in your eyes, flush eyes with plenty of water.

It is suggested to always store hydrogen peroxide away from heat and sunlight. The original solution that was bought should be stored in the freezer for future use.

You must remember that hydrogen peroxide is a caustic substance when used in high concentrations. By diluting it to the proper concentration and not overdosing, it is the key to administering hydrogen peroxide therapy safely, regardless of the application method that you select.

Only 35 Percent "Food Grade" hydrogen peroxide is recommended for internal use. This 35 percent concentration is a very strong oxidizer if it is not diluted and can be extremely dangerous or even fatal. Any concentrations over

10 percent can cause neurological reactions and must be handled carefully because direct contact will burn the skin. Immediate flushing with running water is recommended.

A convenient method of dispensing 35 percent Food Grade hydrogen peroxide is from a small eye dropper bottle, which can be purchased from your Food Grade H_2O_2 distributor or local drugstore. Fill this with your 35 percent Food Grade H_2O_2 and store the larger container in the freezer of your refrigerator for safe keeping until more is needed. The eye dropper bottle can be stored in the refrigerator. The drops are mixed according to the outlined schedule with 6 to 8 ounces of distilled water, natural unsweetened fruit juice, milk, aloe vera juice, or gel.

The generally recommended dosage schedule is outlined in the following chart from a program based on years of experience and reports from thousands of users. Anyone choosing to go at a slower pace can expect slower progress, which is an option. A cumulative effect takes place with each Hydrogen Peroxide treatment by building and enhancing the effects of previous treatments. It is suggested to take the scheduled dosages one hour before eating or 3 hours after eating. If you are taking supplements, you treat them the same as food.

Individuals who have had transplants should not indulge in an H_2O_2 program because H_2O_2 stimulates the immune system and could possibly cause a rejection of the organ. Consult your physician first.

Generally Recommended Dosage Program
Using 35% Food Grade H_2O_2

Day 1	3 drops	3 times daily
Day 2	4 drops	3 times daily
Day 3	5 drops	3 times daily
Day 4	6 drops	3 times daily
Day 5	7 drops	3 times daily
Day 6	8 drops	3 times daily
Day 7	9 drops	3 times daily
Day 8	10 drops	3 times daily
Day 9	12 drops	3 times daily
Day 10	14 drops	3 times daily
Day 11	16 drops	3 times daily
Day 12	18 drops	3 times daily
Day 13	20 drops	3 times daily
Day 14	22 drops	3 times daily
Day 15	24 drops	3 times daily
Day 16	25 drops	3 times daily
Day 17	25 drops	3 times daily
Day 18	25 drops	3 times daily
Day 19	25 drops	3 times daily
Day 20	25 drops	3 times daily
Day 21	25 drops	3 times daily

Suggested After-Dosage Schedule

For more serious complaints, stay at 25 drops 3 times per day for 1 to 3 weeks. Next graduate down to 25 drops, 2 times per day until the problem is taken care of. This may take 1 to 6 months. Don't give up! When free of complaints, you may taper off by using:

25 drops	every other day	4 times
25 drops	every third day	for 2 weeks
25 drops	every fourth day	for 3 weeks

After careful consideration, I managed to purchase 35% food grade hydrogen peroxide (H_2O_2) for my self-administered Hydrogen Peroxide Therapy from a very reliable source, "Guardian of Eden". It is also the largest supplier of 35% food grade H_2O_2 to licensed MD's (medical doctors), clinics, alternative and natural health professionals, water treatment facilities, dairy farms, commercial fruit and berry growers, commercial aquariums, veterinarians, and thousands of individuals for personal use.

Dr. Robert Rowen's Newsletter listed *Guardian of Eden* as a source of 35% food grade hydrogen peroxide. Their website is listed as: Guardian of Eden H_2O_2.

They also sell the more enhanced version of food grade hydrogen peroxide known as Jutran Rx (H_2O_2 and supplements), which consist of hydrogen peroxide supplemented in liquid form with at least 117 protein amino acids and ionized colloidal minerals. It is believed that the hydrogen peroxide breaks down to the most absorbable atomic and molecular level. It also includes adding more oxygen molecules.

Jutran Rx comes in three different grades indicated respectively as: Jutran Rx Brown, Jutran Rx Green, and Jutran Rx Blue. Each of these are packed as a six month supply in two eight ounce bottles made of blue cobalt glass and will last for years in your refrigerator.

Of all of these, the most impressive one appears to be Jutran Rx Blue because it includes pure silver and pure gold, which is broken down to its molecular level to make them more absorbable at that level. Its manufacturing process involves the slow and expensive process of electrolysis. Colloidal silver is rated as one of the most powerful biocides that kill fungus, virus, yeast, etc. Whereby, gold is the best electrical conductor and is believed to assist in the function of the electrical impulses from the nervous system and brain function.

Jutran Rx Blue Part 1 consists of 35% concentration of 100% pure, certified and undiluted food grade hydrogen peroxide. Part 2 consists of the full collection of minerals, amino acids and colloidals, which consist of pure silver, gold or other metal that is broken down into its molecular structure, thereby making it more absorbable at the cellular level.

When Part 1 and Part 2 are mixed together, the hydrogen peroxide breaks down the minerals and amino acids into their molecular level to make them more absorbable. If Part 1 and Part 2 are premixed before use, its interaction builds up pressure, thereby making it difficult to ship it safely in concentrated forms. This may cause bursting of bottles and limiting the concentration levels of minerals and amino acids.

When Part 1 and Part 2 are shipped in two separate bottles and mixed only when ready to use, the levels of minerals, amino acids and colloidals could be increased, thereby making it much more effective than the original Jutran Rx Blue.

This new version of Jutran Rx Blue now has nearly 400% higher concentrations of 117 minerals and amino acids now being offered. Some of which are: Alinine, Amylasse, Antimony, Barium, Beryllium, Bismuth, Boron, Carbonate, Cerium, Choride, Chromium GTF, Cobalt, Copper, Dysprosium, Ellagic Acid, Erbium, Fromide, Fulvic Acid, Galium, Germanium, Gadolinium, Glycine, Colloidal Gold, Histindine, Holmium, Hydrologized collagen, Indium, Iron, Lanthanum, Lipase, Lithium, Magnesium, Maganese, Molybelium, Neodymium, Nickel, Niobium, Nitrogen, Ornithine, Osmium, Palladium, Platinum, Phosphorus, Potassium, Praseodnium, Proline, Quercitin, Rhenium, Rubidium, Samarium, Scandium, Selenium, Serine, Colloidal Silver, Sodium, Strontium, Sulfate, Tantalum,

Taurine, Tellurium, Terbium, Thallium, Tin, Titanium, Tungsten, Tyrosine, Valine, Vanadium, Varium, Yttrium, Ytterblum, Zinc, Zirconium, hydroxproline, L-alinine, L-arginine, L-aspartic acid, L-cysenine,L-glutamic acid, L-Histine, L-hydroxylysine, L-hydroxproline, L-isoleucine. L-Leleucine, L-Lysine, L-methionine, L-phenylaline, L-proline, L-serine, L-threonin, L-tyosine, L-valine, Creatine, ornithine, glutamine, Co-Q6, Co-Q7, Co-Q8, Co-Q10, and fulvic acid.

Neither the FDA nor any other governmental agency has sanctioned benefits from its uses and has not approved or banned hydrogen peroxide usage. Although it was mentioned earlier, the FDA (Food and Drug Administration) has given hydrogen peroxide the GRAS designation (Generally Recognized As Safe), it is advisable to always consult your doctor or health care professional before starting any program.

If you want to find a doctor in your area that is trained in the use of hydrogen peroxide intravenous infusion therapy, contact the International Bio-Oxidative Medicine Foundation (IBOM), P.O. Box 13205, Oklahoma City, Oklahoma 73113. Phone (405) 478-4266.

Chapter 11
Bone Building Nutrient: Strontium

C urrent research reveals that bone fracture risk can be lowered by more than 50 percent by taking the nutrient of natural strontium, which is more effective for bone building than calcium and vitamin D taken together.

Bone density could increase by almost 15 percent in a 3-year period. If you took the more risky conventional therapies over that same 3-year period, you may average an increase of close to half of that, which was achieved by strontium.

Natural strontium should not be mistaken with the manmade substance of strontium-90, which does nothing for bone health. Natural strontium is a safe, non-toxic mineral that helps fragile bones attributed to age, heredity, or other risk factors to eventually become more flexible and stronger thereby helping to reduce your chances of suffering debilitating fractures or even a deadly one.

When strontium was added to women's bone building program, it cut their risk of bone fracture by 49% during the first year. They also increased the bone density in their backs by an average of 14.4% and by 8. 3% in their necks. In comparison, Women who only took calcium and vitamin D didn't see any increase in bone density.

In another study, limiting women from 80 to 100 years of age reduced their risk of fracture by 59% in the first year, by taking strontium.

More studies indicate strontium can help you stand taller with a 20% reduction in the rate of height loss and almost 30% increase in the patients free of back pain.

The research on natural strontium started about 50 years ago at the world famous Mayo Clinic. All of the people who were suffering from severe and painful bone loss that were treated by physicians with strontium had improved.

Even with these surprising results, the potential for bone building by the mineral strontium was silenced for 50 years, possibly because most people believe bone loss is due to a lack of calcium. The dairy industry has billions of dollars at stake in its profits and continually places ads for milk in magazines and airwaves, even though strontium is more effective than calcium for maintaining strong bones.

Strontium is better than calcium because it stimulates rapid formation of bone tissue by acting like a magnet to attract other needed minerals of magnesium, calcium, zinc and boron along with vitamin K-2 to your bones to make them much stronger, and more resistant to fractures, in a relatively short period of time.

Since strontium is denser than calcium, it is more resistant to the cells that break down (osteoclasts). Therefore, it increases your bone density while also resisting bone loss.

Chapter 12
Alzheimer's disease: Cause and Cure

Alzheimer's disease is the most common type of dementia and is the brain disorder named for the well-liked German psychiatrist, Dr. Alois Alzheimer. He was credited for finding the abnormal structures of plaque and tangles in the nerve cells of the brain and published his findings in 1907. After he first described it and drew attention to it, scientists learned a great deal about it as a progressive and fatal brain disease.

A psychiatrist, Dr. Emil Krapelin, was noted for naming and classifying brain disorders, whereas he proposed to name the disease after Alzheimer, which remains to this day.

Alzheimer's destroys brain cells, thereby causing memory loss, problems with thinking and behavior, which could be severe enough to interfere with daily life by affecting work and social life. Over a length of time, Alzheimer's gradually becomes worse and is ultimately fatal.

As our bodies change, our brains also change with most of us noticing slower thinking and problems of memory. It is not a normal part of aging, if our minds are confused and have memory loss. This may be attributed to increasing numbers of brain cells deteriorating and dying.

Research reveals that the Human brain has 100 billion nerve cells (neurons), with each of them communicating with many others and forming more networks. These nerve cell networks have their own special jobs such as remembering, learning and thinking. These networks are also responsible for our vision, hearing, sense of smell, and other senses, while others control our muscular movement.

Dr. Alois Alzheimer discovered the two prime suspects that damage and kill nerve cells are abnormal structures of plaques and tangles. Plaques contain deposits of a protein called beta-amyloid, which builds up between nerve cells. Tangles are formed within the dying nerve cells. As people age, they develop some plaques and tangles. These plaques and tangles appear to form in a predictable manner, first in the areas important for learning, memory, then to other regions. Those afflicted with Alzheimer's develop them much more.

It is believed that plaques and tangles block communication among nerve cells and effectively disrupts the cells activities that are needed to survive. Experts have estimated that 500,000 people between 30 and 50 years-of-age have Alzheimer's or a related dementia.

The average person diagnosed with Alzheimer's lives only about eight years, but others have been known to live with the disease for up to 20 years or more. Presently, more than 5 million Americans are afflicted with Alzheimer's, which is expected to triple by the year of 2050. The mind of an Alzheimer's disease patient could completely vanish from an apparently healthy body, thereby placing his/her total responsibility in the hands of family members, close friends, and other caregivers.

Presently, there is no accepted cure for Alzheimer's disease, current conventional therapies only slow down its progress. Alzheimer's afflicted patients could benefit from taking niacinamide and millions could prevent it by taking 2,000 mg to 3,000 mg a day. It is completely harmless. Studies have shown that a toxic dose in Humans would be about 375,000 mg a day (about 125 times more than the recommended dose). Research indicates that niacinamide is absolutely safe and inexpensive for only about $30 for a possible year's supply.

Niacinamide has a strong effect upon the cells (neurons) in our brain and central nervous system by preventing the buildup of TAU proteins, which form tangles of protein inside of our neurons and prevent normal neural functioning. During the early stages of Alzheimer's, these plump tangles of protein impair nerve cell functions. Ultimately these TAU proteins stop nerve cells from functioning at all and ultimately kill them. Therefore, to prevent Alzheimer's disease and to lessen its effects, these defective TAU proteins should be eliminated from the brain by any means necessary. Niacinamide IS the means by which this can be accomplished.

Niacinamide (vitamin B-3) is a water-soluble vitamin that is quickly absorbed into the bloodstream, causing the levels to begin to rise within about 15 minutes of taking it. It peaks after about 1.5 hours, and then clears itself out of the body after about 3 hours. This appears to be that the maximum effect is achieved by taking 250 mg during every three waking hours, and was considered an ideal maintenance dosage to be taken for life.

William Kaufman, M.D., Ph.D. (1910-2000), was the brilliant nutritionist who had more hands-on experience with niacinamide (vitamin B-3) than anyone. Dr. William Kaufman and his beloved wife, Charlotte, helped him supervise for more than a thousand patient-years by using niacinamide and proving that mental and physical problems of "normal aging" are mostly caused by the shortage of niacinamide in their diets. He was very successful in the use of niacinamide (vitamin B-3) in healing rheumatoid arthritis, osteoarthritis, and other diseases related to vitamin B-3 deficiency.

Dr. Kaufman cured them by prescribing vitamin B-3 up to 4,000 milligrams, divided in 10 doses per day, in a period of one to three months. Dr. Kaufman and his wife, Charlotte, both took 250 mg every three hours for a total of 1,500 mg of niacinamide each day over an 18-hour period for 55 years. Also, based on Dr. Kaufman's studies, it appeared that Alzheimer's patients achieved the best results by taking 250 mg every 1½ hours for 12 doses.

If you or a loved one is afflicted with rheumatic arthritis, osteoarthritis, impaired joint mobility and desire to use niacinamide, it would be a wise decision to also take a whey type of protein to also help furnish the adequate amount of protein to help joint repair. Since cartilage is high in protein, it cannot repair itself without it.

When Dr. Kaufman began his career in the 1940's, Alzheimer's disease never became a focus of his work because it wasn't a common problem. He and his wife, Charlotte, were a perfect team for over 60 years and kept finding in more detail the effects of niacinamide, their dosages, their frequency, and their respective results.

Niacinamide (Nicotinic Acid) is a gentler form of niacin, which is also called vitamin B-3. It protects brains from further memory loss and restores lost memory function for Alzheimer's disease victims. If you are over 65 years of age, there is a one-chance-in-ten that you already have Alzheimer's disease.

Niacinamide has an open-door entrance to the central

nervous system and has a strong attraction for the nervous system's benzodiazepine receptors, thereby causing a pleasant calming effect. It also improves central nervous system function in central nervous system impairments and is a systemic therapeutic agent. It improves muscle strength, joint mobility, decreases fatigue, reduces and eliminates arthritic joint pain. Niacinamide also heals broken strands of DNA and improves many kinds of Central Nervous System functions.

Dr. William Kaufman died at 88 years of age in year 2000 and his wife also passed away at 87 years of age in 2005, only three years short of the California discovery of her life long work with the mysteries of niacinamide, which could be used to save possibly a hundred million lives, especially those afflicted with Alzheimer's disease.

Dr. Alois Alzheimer was credited with the discovery of Alzheimer's disease. Dr. William Kaufman was credited with discovering the power of niacinamide. Dr. Kim N. Green, Ph.D. and his partner Dr. Frank La Perla, of the Department of Neurology and Behavior at University of California at Irvine, became the new heroes of Alzheimer's disease research.

Dr. Kim Green arrived at the 1,000 to 3,000 milligram vitamin B-3 schedule by actually witnessing the response of patients with varying degrees of arthritis. He could not give a single large dose of 2,000 to 3,000 milligram of niacinamide and get any favorable results.

It was necessary to divide the doses to keep the blood levels of niacinamide uniform throughout the day. The 250 mg. niacinamide thin gelatin capsules were more efficient for delivery in the treatment of joint dysfunction (arthritis) and were taken in separate doses throughout the day to add up to the total of 2,000 to 3,000 mg per day.

Dr. Kim Green headed a four-month study of a treatment for Alzheimer's disease equivalent to 2,000 to 3,000 milligrams of niacinamide per day in divided doses. Dr. Green said, "Cognitively, they were cured. The vitamin completely prevented cognitive decline associated with the disease, bringing them back to the level they'd be at if they didn't have the pathology.

Dr. Green explains: "Microtubules are like highways inside cells. What we're doing with nicotinamide is making a wider, more stable highway. In Alzheimer's disease, this highway breaks down. We are preventing this from happening."

Niacinamide also works by removing "tangles" of a bad protein in brain cells referred to as TAU. Within Alzheimer's disease patients, the protein becomes poisonous and also contributes to dangerous clogging within the brain's nerve cells.

Our bodies' own stress hormone production raises production of the beta-amyloid protein production, which causes waxy clumps of plaque to build up in the brain cells. This can easily be the reason why younger people from 30 to 50 years of age are also being afflicted with Alzheimer's disease.

If you or anyone you know has any noticeable symptoms of Alzheimer's or any other form of dementia, it should be considered to take 1500 mg twice daily. You can save and normalize Alzheimer's disease and its associated dementia with niacinamide (vitamin B-3).

Those brain-clogging plaques and tangles were formed over many years, therefore they're not likely to dissolve in a few hours. Niacinamide is said to work miracles, but it doesn't erase all the damage instantly. Niacinamide can be found at a health food store and on the Internet.

Niacinamide has been used for over 20 years with amazing improvements in patients' muscle weakness, mobility problems, sense of balance, osteoarthritis, and fatigue. Even if you are an average person, it also improves memory, behavior, and makes you better than you are now.

The beneficial impacts of niacinamide may be multiplied by also taking one or more of these supplements: curcumin, lecithin, alpha lipoic acid, acetyl choline, acetyl-L-carnitine, silymarin, galantamide, and/or reservatrol.

At present, it is believed that millions of Alzheimers' sufferers could benefit from high doses of niacinamide and many more could possibly prevent it by taking it.

There are no negative side effects of niacinamide supplementation and it has never been reported as a cause of death or cause of "liver damage." Compare this to the well-meaning M.D.s' that cause more than 250,000 deaths each year by their "properly prescribed" drugs.

Chapter 13
Earliest Diagnosis of Cancer:
The AMAS Test

Presently, more than one of every three of us will contract Cancer and may very well be 1-in-2 of us during our lifetime. Therefore, I sincerely believe that the importance of taking the AMAS (Anti-Malignan Antibody in Serum test should be stressed upon again, from a chapter of my first book "Win the Ultimate Battle for Your Health".

In 1974, a Harvard-trained research chemist, Samuel Boguch, MD, PhD, and his researcher wife, Eleanor Boguch, MD, discovered a new antigen that was located on all cancer cells. Apparently, when the cancer cells bump into each other, the outer layer is ground off and exposes the inner protein layer and the malignant antigen. When the body's immune system identifies this foreign protein, as not part of the body's normal biology, it produces antibodies to destroy it.

In 1992, Dr. Samuel Boguch and his wife Eleanor were two research scientists at Boston Medical School, who devised the AMAS blood test to measure the antibodies within our body in response to early cancer. The cell-surface that is found to be present on all malignant cells was thereby given the name of "malignan". The AMAS (Anti-Malignan Antibody in Serum) test detects the anti-malignan in the blood.

This valuable blood test aids in detecting, diagnosing, and monitoring of malignant cancer present anywhere within the human body and was first made available in the United States through Oncolab Inc. Since 1977, it has established an excellent track record over many years. Oncolab is the laboratory that was founded in Boston, Massachusetts for research and and clinical purposes by Dr. Samuel Boguch, MD, PhD, a Harvard-trained research neurochemist and his researcher wife, Eleanor Boguch, MD. Clinical trials were performed with more than 4,000 patients over a seven-year period, thereby validating the AMAS test's effectiveness.

The AMAS test does not look for cancer antigens in the blood stream. That condition generally arises when a specific late-stage and relatively large malignant tumor mass (of about 1 billion malignant cells) is already present as a metastatic disease. But the AMAS test does measure the level of certain anti-cancer antibodies within the blood serum. Therefore, this measurement of selecting specific anti-cancer antibodies means that the AMAS test may be very helpful in the early detection of relatively small numbers of malignant cancer cells within the body. These could appear at least 19 months earlier, and before they can be discovered as a malignant tumor mass with an MRI, CT scan or many of the other cancer blood tests that are currently being used. But the MRI, CT scan and other conventional medicine's cancer blood tests can not be a positive indication of a malignant tumor without additional expensive tests.

The American and Canadian Societies realize that early detection of cancer can bring on early treatment of defeating cancer and reduce its harmful effects. After the "clinical cancer" has been identified with the AMAS test, specific anti-cancer treatments could be started and the AMAS test could be used to monitor the treatment progress of the ongoing therapy.

Dr. Boguch and his colleagues studied abnormally high serum AMA levels that were greater than 134 micrograms per milliliter of blood and were discovered to be a usual appearance of all types of malignancies. This Anti-Malignan Antibody (AMA) presence in blood serum serves as a marker of malignant transformation by converting normal body cells to cancerous cells. During the process, the AMA is a type of anti-body produced by the body's immune system, which becomes present in the blood and extracellular fluid. The AMA binds itself to a cell-surface protein which is the antigen that is present on malignant cancer cells, whereby this antigen was given the name of "malignan".

The malignan is measured within the plasma membranes of malignant tumor cells, but the test cannot find any malignan within the membranes of normal cells or benign tumor cells because there does not appear to be any to be measured. The reason could be that the cell's biochemistry shifts during the malignant transformation from aerobic metabolism (requiring oxygen) to anaerobic metabolism (not requiring oxygen). In other words, the process shifts from the respiration process of oxygen taking place within normal aerobic cells to the fermentation process, which takes place in the absence of oxygen within the cancer cells anaerobic metabolism.

When the AMAS test results show 100-134 micrograms of antigens per milliliter of blood, it is considered borderline. But when the test shows 135 micrograms of antigens or more per milliliter of blood, it is considered as "clinical cancer". Clinically cancer-free "normal" people always have small numbers of malignantly transformed cells present in their bodies because their immune system does a terrific job of eliminating them. But you can't ever get to an antigen count of zero. Therefore, it is always essential to maintain a good strong immune system.

Your body's AMA appears to be very important as an anti-cancer immune surveillance system. After your AMA rises above 134 micrograms per milliliter of blood, you have "clinical cancer". After this, you can start successful anti-cancer therapeutic intervention with immune therapy, cytotoxic drug therapy, radiation, surgery, etc. After therapy begins, the AMAS test can be taken again in three more months to monitor progress and see if the AMA in the blood has lowered below the cancer level of 135 mcg/ml and lower. Even though 100mcg/ml and up to 134 mcg/ml is considered "border line", these results are seen in normal individuals and cancer patients who are successfully treated and are in remission from "clinical cancer".

False negatives may be observed in advanced terminally ill cancer patients who are in a state of "antibody failure" due to disease-induced immune suppression. That means these individuals have a depleted immune system and are no longer able to synthesize sufficient amounts of cancer fighting cells and antibodies such as the AMA.

Oncologists are experienced medical professionals that can usually distinguish the four clinical states by their overall clinical picture of the patient, such as: an active cancer state, the advanced terminal/cancer state, the successfully-treated remission state, and the normal non-cancer state. It is possible to distinguish between advanced or terminal cancer patients who show apparently normal AMAS levels from the successfully-treated cancer patients in remission who show normal AMAS test values. This clinical determination is based upon the physician's clinical oncology experience. Additional AMAS tests and monitoring may be necessary in uncertain cases.

The AMAS test is highly sensitive and highly accurate with high specificity based on published scientific papers. The US Food and Drug Administration gave Dr. Boguch "permission to market" the AMAS test with the following FDA approved statements: "If repeat determinations agree, the false-positive and false-negative rates are less than 1% (Specificity and sensitivity greater than 99%) ; in single determinations, false positives are 5% and false negatives are 7% (3,315 double-blind tests of patients and controls)".

These low rates mean that the AMAS test appears as a superior diagnostic for malignant cancer when compared with any other currently available tests, which are only useful in late-stage cancer detection involving large tumor masses or multiple metastases and often show high false negative rates during early stages of "clinical cancer". Tests other than the AMAS test also show high positive rates in various benign neoplastic and non-neoplastic disorders and physiological states. Therefore, these tests contain errors in a diagnosis of malignant cancer.

If you or any of your loved ones are interested in taking

the AMAS test, call Oncolab before 6 P.M. Eastern Time at (800) 922-8378 or (617 536-0850. The AMAS kit is free but the current cost of processing an AMAS test is $135. (US).

Oncolab does not pay for blood separation of the serum, shipping by overnight FEDEX morning delivery, nor the costs of blood drawing (phlebotomy). You can also visit "AMAS Cancer TEST.Com" on the Internet. Medicare and other insurances pay for it in some plans, CPT (billing) code 86-317. The AMAS test has been patented by the U.S. Government and is FDA approved. Oncolab accepts Medicare as full payment.

After you have received your AMAS test kit, you must obtain a doctor's signature to approve your blood test. Then schedule your blood test between Monday and Thursday. Smith Kline and Lab Corp are familiar with specifications of drawing blood for Oncolab's AMAS test and may also be able to arrange for shipping as well.

Since your doctor's fax number is on the authorization form, results could be received in as few as three to seven days.

The AMAS test is a blood test that measures the amount of anti-malignan antibodies in the blood, which is based on measurements of S-TAG, F-TAG, Net-TAG and its interpretation. To receive the "Overall Results", subtract F-TAG results from the S-TAG results, which will then give you the Net-TAG. This Net TAG result measures the

117

antibody count in micrograms per milliliter. The antibody count can be detected about 19 months earlier than the antigens (associated with cancer), thereby allowing you about a 19 month head start to treat your cancer.

Chapter 14
Our Conventional Medical
& Pharmaceutical Professions

Presently, the medical and pharmaceutical professions in the United States are a thriving one trillion dollar a year business. Pharmaceutical companies have manufactured and promoted medical "breakthroughs" and "miracle drugs", which have never prevented or cured any diseases. Americans can anticipate spending a total of more than $3 trillion dollars within the next 10 years during which time more than $1 trillion dollars is anticipated to be spent on drugs. Can you see why the pharmaceutical industry has no incentive to keep us in good health when it is currently THE most profitable industry in the world?

The Pharmaceutical Industry has huge profit margins

on its drugs that can variously yield up to 50,000 percent; and some drugs have even greater than 500,000 percent markups. The pharmaceutical industry manufactures drugs to only treat symptoms but not to cure diseases. Therefore, they have more to gain when we remain sick... by KEEP-ING us sick... rather than having us get well.

The Pharmaceutical Industry has great power with their unlimited financial resources to keep doctors from prescribing natural therapies. They have established a pharmaceutical cartel of lobbyists that outnumber con-gressmen by two-to-one with about $100 million spent an-nually to protect its profits. They have succeeded in influ-encing congress to disallow health claims for natural rem-edies. They also spent huge amounts of money through their drug commercials in order to convince the American public in believing that they have a health problem and to have the doctors prescribe their drugs to patients. They have deceived millions of people through their elaborate control of manipulation and economic incentives to de-ceive people into believing that drugs are the only answer to disease. That just goes to show you, if someone lies often enough people are going to believe it.

The FDA (Food and Drug Administration) is the gov-ernment agency that was created to protect public health. Nevertheless, many of the FDA's senior management and members of its advisory committee accept generous amounts of money in corporate grants, contracts and consulting fees from pharmaceutical companies. As if this is not enough, some of the FDA officials have been rewarded with pharmaceutical company jobs upon leaving their positions with the FDA.

A former FDA investigator exposed aspartame (artificial sweetener) as a deadly neurotoxin. The "revolving door" at the FDA is very much a reality. Former corporate officials who began working for the Food and Drug Administration (and vice versa), were very arrogant about issues uncovered at the G. D. Searle laboratory surrounding their drug processing and issues involved with aspartame. Some of them had a hidden agenda of promised secret money or better jobs, which actively hindered the investigation into G. D. Searle's laboratory practices.

It would be obvious to us if we were able to see the records and numbers and where those jobs were. These are a matter of public and Congressional Record. Subsequently, many former FDA officials, due to their "favorable influences" with regulatory enforcement and rulings, were in fact, rewarded with corporate positions and lucrative incomes, including former FDA Commissioner Arthur Hull Hayes, who was about to be brought up on ethics and misconduct charges.

Dr. Herbert Ley, former FDA commissioner was quoted as follows, "The thing that bugs me is that people think the FDA (Food and Drug Administration) is protecting them. It is not. What the FDA is doing and what the public thinks it's doing are as different as night and day."

Dr. James P. Carter, M. D., author of *Racketeering In Medicine: The Suppression of Alternatives*, was quoted as follows, "The FDA serves as the pharmaceutical industry's watchdog, which can be called upon to attack and destroy a potential competitor under the guise of protecting the public."

The Washington Times reported top scientists at the FDA have financial conflicts of interest regarding drugs that come under their scrutiny. These are often tied up in the form of stock options, which are commonly waived and hidden from the public. Many of the scientists are under pressure to recommend approval of a new drug even if they have reservations about its safety or its effectiveness. This process has been going on for years and the results continue to be disastrous with their "approved" drugs killing more than 100,000 people each year. Therefore, the FDA has failed entirely in its mandate to be the primary custodian responsible for our national health.

In 1992, researchers at Harvard discovered there were approval deadlines that were imposed on the FDA by Congress because pharmaceutical companies agreed to pay millions of dollars in fees to the FDA to help their inefficient agency in hiring more reviewers to help clear the abundance of drug applications. This revealed that a disturbing relationship existed with the drugs that received ultra-fast FDA approvals and the drugs that needed to be pulled off the market due to safety issues.

The FDA agreed to speed the approval or rejection of 90 percent of all drugs within a year of the applications' submissions, or the millions in fees would be refunded by the FDA. "High Priority" drugs or lifesaving drugs are to be approved by the FDA in only six months.

It appears outrageous that the Food and Drug Administration (FDA) enters into a lucrative financial arrangement with the same pharmaceutical companies of whose drugs they were meant to monitor and review the safety of the food and drugs for public consumption. The FDA appears to be a government agency that does not want to be giving back money, once a possible refund is likely. Therefore, the FDA is urged into action and is more likely to approve a drug in two months leading up to a deadline.

Dr. Steve Nissen, chief of cardiology of the Cleveland Clinic was among the first to be concerned with drugs such as Vioxx, Rozullin, Bextra and Baycol (Bayer's statin drug). Coincidently, they were all approved in time to meet their approval date and were ultimately taken off the market, after the loss of many lives. This may be referred to as a wake-up call that places the FDA in a difficult position under very tight deadlines to make complex decisions.

There definitely appears to be a serious conflict of interest by the FDA when it approves the drugs fast in order not to lose the millions in fees paid by the pharmaceutical industry. Even if the FDA has the option of denying approval of a drug due to safety concerns, they are not likely to do so.

Just recently, twenty percent or 200 of the nearly 1,000 scientists working for the FDA said they were asked by the heads of the FDA to provide incomplete and inaccurate misleading information. There are probably hundreds more in this group of scientists that did not confess to being requested to perform deceitful acts.

It appears that the pharmaceutical industry has been responsible for hundreds of thousands of deaths over the years, and perhaps even millions. The pharmaceutical companies are going to Supreme Court in order to instate a preemption policy involving the FDA. In their lawsuit, the companies are essentially saying that: Since the FDA approved each drug before it was released to the market, the FDA was satisfied and the pharmaceutical companies shouldn't be held liable for any damages. If the courts rule against this, it means the courts are overruling the FDA, whom already gave their approval for the drug.

Since it appears that the FDA only finds out very little of all serious adverse reactions to drugs, it cannot possibly guarantee the drug's safety and protect the public's interest.

It is also interesting to know, the studies, which are needed to gain drug approval by the FDA are short, and are usually conducted by the pharmaceutical manufacturer.

It was reported by the *New York Times* that oncologists

(cancer-treating medical specialists) are being paid kick-backs by the pharmaceutical companies in order to prescribe their questionable drugs. An oncology group of six doctors received $2.7 million in kickbacks for prescribing $9 million worth of its drugs in only one year.

The cancer drug Avastin (Bevacizuman) was first introduced in the United States, as its first market by the pharmaceutical giant, Roche. This was accomplished with the help of our government, through our tax dollars, by sponsoring the drug's research, which eventually helped it to receive a patent.

Roche's U. S. government sponsored trial of the drug was started in early 2005 in the United Kingdom, Germany, and Switzerland. It is also interesting to note, after receiving their patent, Roche and Guenentech (its co-developer of Avastin) were at liberty to name their own price of the drug. Guenentech priced the Avastin drug at $4,400 a month at first, which was about $1,000 more than its price in the United Kingdom. Avastin could cost anywhere from $4,400 to $8,800 a month, depending on the treatment. According to the *New York Times*, February 15, 2006, a year's cancer treatment with Avastin costs $100,000. Some desperate patients have been known to pay for their treatments by mortgaging their homes and even going broke in order to stay alive.

If American progress is based upon developing new drugs to fight disease, we as taxpayers pay for it in two basic ways... As taxpayers, we support the research through the National Institutes of Health (NIH) and through federal tax deductions on Research and Development (R&D) costs of the pharmaceutical industry. As consumers, we support research and development by paying their high prices made possible by their exclusive patents from the government granted monopolies that rewarded their innovative drug.

Most conventional cancer treatments are a miserable failure but the cancer industry tries everything to continue their use and discourage treatments that do not involve drugs, radiation, or surgery, and keep them away from you.

Alan C. Nixon, PhD, former president of the American Chemical Society, as a chemist trained to interpret data, mentioned that chemotherapy does much more harm than good. What does this tell you about any benefits obtained by a cancer patient undergoing chemotherapy?

On Wednesday September 4, 2009, Federal prosecutors accused the world's largest drug maker (Pfizer) of being a repeat corporate cheat for illegal drug promotions and won a record-breaking $2.3 billion in fines. The $1.2 billion criminal fine was the largest of any U.S. criminal case. The total fine included $1 billion in civil penalties and a $100 million criminal forfeiture.

Authorities mentioned Pfizer was a repeat offender and has settled government charges for the fourth time in the last 10 years. The allegations were centered on the marketing of 13 different drugs, which included their big sellers such as Lipitor, Viagra, and Zoloft. Our government said Pfizer also paid kickbacks to market big name drugs: Aricept, Celebrex, Lipitor, Norvac, Ralpax, Viagra, Zithromax, Zoloft and Zyntec.

Mike Loucks, the U. S. attorney in Massachusetts said Pfizer was continuing to violate the same laws with other drugs, even as Pfizer was negotiating deals on their past misconduct.

The settlement also resulted in guilty pleas from two former Pfizer sales managers that resulted in ending the investigation. Even though the drug industry has paid out more than $11 billion in such settlements over the past 19 years, it may not be likely to curb their abuses.

Bill Vaughan, an analyst at Consumers Union, which is a non-profit publisher of Consumer Reports said, "There's so much money in selling pills that there is a tremendous temptation to cheat. There's a kind of mentality in this sector that [settlements] are a cost of doing business and we can cheat. This penalty is so huge I think consumers can have some hope that maybe these guys will tighten up and run a better ship." My guess is that, since people are creatures of habit, the cheating habit is not likely to change.

Dr. Julie Gerberding, former head of the CDC (Centers for Disease Control) U. S. Government agency from 2002-2009 has landed a very lucrative job with Merck as the new president of its vaccine division. Since she is now heading a $5 billion vaccine industry, she is probably earning at least 10 times more than our own president of the United States.

For years while Dr. Gerberding was head of the CDC, she was defending Merck's vaccines and maintained the position that Merck's vaccines are so safe that all side effects should be dismissed. It could make a person wonder whether there was some ongoing collusion between Merck and the CDC and to what degree Dr. Gerberding may have been involved.

Dr. Gerberding admitted that vaccines can cause Autism-like symptoms to be exactly the same as the symptoms that define Autism disease. What does this tell you?

Bibliography:
References Cited and
Sources of Further Information

These are some of the resources that I have read, consulted, or referred to both directly and indirectly during the writing of this book. I recommend these resources to you the reader for more detailed information on any of the topics that have been so briefly touched upon herein. This book and these further resources will give you a good fighting start in doing your own research and in taking personal control and responsibility for winning the ultimate battle for your health. Best Wishes, Good Luck, and Good Health to You!

Balch, James and Stengler, Mark. 2004. *Prescription for Natural Cures: A Self-Care Guide for Treating Health*

Problems with Natural Remedies Including Diet and Nutrition, Nutritional Supplements, Bodywork, and More. Hoboken, NJ. 736 p.

Balch, J. (Ed.) (monthly newsletter). Dr. James Balch's *"Live Well Naturally Newsletter"*. www.LiveWellNaturally.com.

Batmanghelidj, F. 1995. *Your Body's Many Cries for Water: Second Edition.* Vienna, VA: Global Health Solutions; 182 p.

Brooks, T.J. 1963. *Essentials of Medical Parasitology.* New York, NY: McMillan & Company. 1963. 358 p.

Carter, J.P. *Racketeering in Medicine: The Suppression of Alternatives*, Charlottesville, VA: Hampton Roads Publishing Company, Inc. 1993. 392 p.

Clark, H.R. 1993. *The Cure for All Cancers: Including Over 100 Case Histories of Persons Cured.* San Diego, CA: ProMotion Publishers. 1993.

Clark, H.R. 1995. *The Cure for All Diseases: With Many case Histories.* San Diego, CA: New Century Press. 1995.

Clark, H.R (Website) Hulda Regehr Clark Information Center: www.DrClark.com

Douglass, W.C. (Ed.) Real Health Breakthroughs (monthly newsletter). Dr. William Campbell Douglass. *The Douglass Report.* www.DouglassReport.com.

Duarte, Alex. 1995. *Dr. Duarte's Health Alternatives: Your Exclusive Health Management System* by Alex Duarte Publisher: Morton Grove, IL.: Mega Systems Inc. 1995; Audio Cassette Set With Book. 16 Audio Cassette Tapes and book 444 p.

Fischer, D.S., Knobf, M.T., Durivage, H.J., & Beaulieu, N.J. *The Cancer Chemotherapy Handbook (6th Edition).* Philadelphia, PA: Mosby. 2003. 640 p.

Jensen, Bernard. 2000. *Dr. Jensen's Guide to Diet and Detoxification: Healthy Secrets from Around the World.* Lincolnwood, IL: Keats Publishing. 128 p.

Langsjoen, P.H., Folkers, K. 1993. Isolated diastolic dysfunction of the myocardium and its response to CoQ10 treatment. In: *Seventh International Symposium on Biomedical and Clinical Aspects of Coenzyme Q.* In: Folkers, K., Mortensen, S.A., Littarru, G.P., Yamagami, T., and Lenaz, G. (eds) *The Clinical Investigator,* 1993. 71:S140-S144.

Life Extension. (monthly newsletter). www.LEF.org

McDougall, J.A. (Ed.) (monthly newsletter). Dr. John A. McDougall's *"To Your Health"* www.DrMcDougall.com.

Rowen, R.J. (Ed.) (monthly newsletter). Dr. Robert J. Rowen's *Second Opinion.* www.SecondOpinionNewsletter. com.

Sinatra, S. (Ed.) (monthly newsletter). Dr. Steven Sinatra's *"Heart, Health & Nutrition".* www.DrSinatra.com.

Tasseff, Thomas. 2008. **Win the Ultimate Battle for your Health: The Lifesaving Legacy of Tom Tasseff.** Denver, Colorado: Outskirts Press. 2008. 236 p. Available in Hardcover, Softcover, and Digital Media. www.OutskirtsPress. com; Amazon.com; Barnes & Noble Booksellers; and at a bookstore near you. ISBN# 978-1-4327-2796-3.

Thompson, J. (Ed.) (monthly newsletter). Dr. Jenny Thompson. *Health Sciences Institute Newsletter.* www. HSIBaltimore.com

Torrey, E.F. 1983. *Surviving Schizophrenia: A Manual for Families, Consumers, and Providers (4th Edition).* New York, NY: Harper Collins Publishers, Inc. 544 p.

Torrey, E.F. 1984. *The Roots of Treason: Ezra Pound and the Secret of St. Elizabeth's*. 1984. London: Sidgwick & Jackson

USA Today, January 11, 1999 America's Goo And Glue Diet.

Weinberger, Stanley. 1993. *Parasites: An Epidemic in Disguise.* Healing Within Products. 58 p.

West, B. (Ed.) (monthly newsletter). Dr. Bruce West's "*Health Alert*". www.HealthAlert.com.

Whitaker, J. (Ed.) (monthly newsletter). *Health & Healing: Tomorrow's Medicine Today.* www.DrWhitaker.com.

Williams, D. (Ed.) (monthly newsletter). Dr. David William's *Alternatives for the Health Conscious Individual.* www.DrDavidWilliams.com

Postscript

This book was written in my eightieth year of life to share with you new information that has come to light since the publication of my first book *Win the Ultimate Battle for your Health: The Lifesaving Legacy of Tom Tasseff* (Outskirts Press 2008; Amazon.com; Barnes & Noble). Although each book stands alone perfectly well in its respective lifesaving strategies, I strongly recommend that you obtain a copy of my earlier work at once and keep both of these books in your arsenal of lifesaving literature. Together they provide you the means to a longer, happier, and healthier life... my continuing legacy to you!

My intention in writing this book is to share with you what I have learned and employed in winning the ultimate battle for my own health as based upon a lifetime of good living, from conducting my own in-depth research, and from the experience of overcoming my own health obstacles. My legacy to you is to provide you with the ammunition that I have found available and have used to improve my own general health and happiness.

It is my hope that as you read this book, you will do so with an open mind and find both the information and the inspiration to continue to do your own research, to seek appropriate and cooperative professional medical health care consultation as necessary, and to make informed decisions that will lead you to a healthier and happier life.

None of the information provided nor any of the opinions expressed in this publication should be construed as personal medical advice or instruction. No action should be taken based solely upon on the contents of this book. Readers are advised to consult their own appropriate health care professionals on any matters relating to their personal medical health, health concerns, symptoms, illness, disease, or treatment strategies. This means... "See Your Doctor."

No information contained herein, as expressed, or as implied, or as might be interpreted by the reader, is intended to diagnose, treat, cure, or prevent any disease. That is why the reader is advised again to seek his or her own personal professional medical consultation. I have done my very best to ensure that the contents of this book are accurate. The information contained herein is based upon my own personal research and personal experience and while I believe it to be correct and accurate as based entirely upon my own research and experience, it cannot be guaranteed in any way to be correct and accurate. No warrantee or guarantee of any kind is stated, intended, expressed, or implied.

While the information provided and the opinions expressed in this book are believed to be accurate and are based on the best judgment of the author, readers who fail to consult with appropriate health care authorities assume ALL risk for ANY injury and for consequences of any kind. Neither the author, nor the publisher, nor any person associated with the writing, editing, publication, printing, or distribution of this book is liable for any errors, inaccuracies, or omissions. The reader assumes ALL responsibility for ANY actions taken and is repeatedly advised to seek appropriate professional medical consultation.

Neither the U.S. Food and Drug Administration (USF-DA) nor the American Medical Association (AMA) have approved any of the materials contained, practices described, or information presented in this book. The author does however recommend that the USFDA, the AMA, medicine, big medicine, big drug and pharmaceutical companies, and big money finally admit to us the benefits of natural and herbal remedies, which can quickly and cost effectively save millions of our dollars and both prolong and save millions of our lives each year.

About The Author

Tom Tasseff was born to Macedonian parents in the "Steel City", Lackawanna, New York on April 10, 1931. He was the eldest son and the third of seven children. His proud Eastern European family traditions and upbringing during both the Great Depression and the Second World War contributed greatly to his success, his patriotism, and his strong American work ethic.

During World War II when Tom was only twelve years old, he supplemented his family income by working as a shoe-shine boy. It was at this time that he bought his first fitness magazine, *Strength & Health*, which featured articles by the magazine's editor Bob Hoffman as well as John Grimek, Steve Stanko, and many other early fitness gurus. As Tom's collection of *Strength & Health* magazines accumulated, he was encouraged and inspired by the monthly features and learned to develop good health habits to maintain a "sound mind and a healthy body".

After graduating from Lackawanna High School in 1950, he went to work at Bethlehem Steel, earning and saving enough money to attend classes at Canisius College in nearby Buffalo, New York. However, it was then that his nation called him to service during the Korean War. Tom was activated into the U.S. Navy Air Corps in which he was already proudly serving as a reservist.

Once activated in the Navy, Tom was fortunate enough to attend the training school of his choice because of his very high scores on the Navy Achievement Tests. He successfully completed his Aerology-Meteorology training in Lakehurst, New Jersey and served as a U.S. Navy Weatherman for four years during the Korean War. Tom received an honorable discharge in 1955 from his final base of operations at the U.S. Naval Air Station in Columbus, Ohio. Upon Tom's discharge from the Navy, he went back to work at Bethlehem Steel as a trouble- shooting electrician for diversified electrical controls in the Blast Furnace Department until the steel plant's shutdown in 1983.

Not willing to become another casualty of "The Rust Belt", Tom focused his attention, his hard-earned assets, and his ingenuity on becoming a builder of homes and a developer of residential subdivisions. Tom's first subdivision was Tasseff Terrace in Hamburg, New York where he built a home for Russell "Rusty" Jones, the physical conditioning coach of the Buffalo Bills Football team. They remained good friends and neighbors until Rusty moved to Chicago in 2004 to become the physical conditioning coach of the Chicago Bears.

After building Tasseff Terrace Subdivision, Tom built the nearby Ridgefield Estates Subdivision and has most recently completed the scenic Castle Ridge Subdivision all in the lovely and quaint little Town of Hamburg, New York where Tom and his dear wife, Nada, currently reside.

Throughout his life, Tom Tasseff has continued his research on health, fitness, and the prevention of disease. He attributes much of his personal and professional success to his healthy body and his healthy mind. He wrote this book to share with you what he has learned and employed over his lifetime in hopes that you too will be encouraged to take positive action and take responsibility for and control of your life, your health, your happiness, and your destiny.

Other Books By Tom Tasseff:

Win the Ultimate Battle for your Health: The Lifesaving Legacy of Tom Tasseff. Outskirts Press: Denver, Colorado. 2008. 236 Pages.

CPSIA information can be obtained at www.ICGtesting.com
Printed in the USA
BVOW05s1705080215

386734BV00001B/37/P

9 781432 762407